T0367555

Healthy
Tipping
Point

AVERY

a member of

Penguin Group (USA) Inc.

New York

Healthy Tipping Point

A POWERFUL PROGRAM FOR A STRONGER, HAPPIER YOU

Caitlin Boyle

Published by the Penguin Group
Penguin Group (USA) Inc., 375 Hudson Street, New York, New York 10014, USA •
Penguin Group (Canada), 90 Eglinton Avenue East, Suite 700, Toronto, Ontario M4P 2Y3,
Canada (a division of Pearson Penguin Canada Inc.) • Penguin Books Ltd, 80 Strand, London WC2R 0RL,
England • Penguin Ireland, 25 St Stephen's Green, Dublin 2, Ireland (a division of Penguin Books Ltd) •
Penguin Group (Australia), 250 Camberwell Road, Camberwell, Victoria 3124, Australia (a division of
Pearson Australia Group Pty Ltd) • Penguin Books India Pvt Ltd, 11 Community Centre, Panchsheel Park,
New Delhi–110 017, India • Penguin Group (NZ), 67 Apollo Drive, Rosedale, North Shore 0632,
New Zealand (a division of Pearson New Zealand Ltd) • Penguin Books (South Africa) (Pty) Ltd,
24 Sturdee Avenue, Rosebank, Johannesburg 2196, South Africa

Penguin Books Ltd, Registered Offices: 80 Strand, London WC2R 0RL, England

Library of Congress Cataloging-in-Publication Data
Boyle, Caitlin.
Healthy tipping point : a powerful program for a stronger, happier you / Caitlin Boyle.
p.   cm.
ISBN 978-1-58333-496-6
1. Self-care, Health.   2. Nutrition.   3. Physical fitness.   I. Title.
RA776.95.B69   2012   2011052356
613—dc23

Book design by Meighan Cavanaugh

ALWAYS LEARNING   PEARSON

To Lauren,

a true friend who encouraged me

to begin this journey

Contents

Part I
GET REAL

Part II

EAT CLEAN

Part III

EMBRACE STRENGTH

Part IV

CONCLUSION

INTRODUCTION:
A HOLISTIC HEALTHY
TIPPING POINT

There's living, and then there's being *alive*.

Many people spend their whole life merely . . . existing. They're haunted by a dull, sinking feeling that they're constantly sprinting, running as hard as they can, and yet standing perfectly still—getting nowhere fast. Perhaps that's why you're reading this book in the first place— you feel emotionally or physically stuck.

For a long time, I felt stuck, too. More often than not, I felt like I was watching my own life from a distance, entirely disconnected from any larger sense of purpose. I was simply going through the motions of my life, checking off boxes that I wasn't sure I even wanted. I went to work to pay the bills, I hit up happy hour for the same old conversations, I came home and watched reality television until brain rot set in, and then I went to sleep. Wake up, caffeinate, and repeat. That terrible sense of sprinting in place oozed over me like thick, hot mud. In a mess of unhealthy habits and negative coping mechanisms, I lost myself.

It's easy to think that being truly alive is marked by muscles and clear skin, a taut stomach and white teeth, and eight hours of perfectly blissful sleep every night. You know—all the physical hallmarks of health that have been pounded into our brains by diet books and fitness magazines for years and years. When you feel as I did—emotionally and physically stuck—it's natural to think that working on the outside will resolve all the messy emotions on the inside, too. If you could just get the physical side of your life under control, the emotional side will follow suit and for once—finally!—you'll feel happy, satisfied, and alive . . . right?

Most diet books play on our belief that the sole way to a healthy, happy, and balanced life is via a perfect appearance. According to *that* type of diet book, this requires the right combination of food and exercise gimmicks and, of course, sheer willpower. You don't have to worry about messy emotions at all; it's just a matter of calorie counting, not eating after six o'clock, eating only green food, not eating white foods, avoiding dairy, inhaling protein, shunning carbohydrates, or simply sticking to the latest and greatest diet fad. Sure, the method sounds a little nuts and a whole lot restrictive. Sure, you'd rather die than reveal your tactics to a friend, who will undoubtedly roll her eyes and say, "Are you serious?" And yes, if pressed, you'd admit there's no way you'd be able to maintain this diet for six months, let alone a lifetime.

And yet many of us keep buying into this philosophy over and over again, despite the fact that it is filled with half promises and only addresses *part* of one side of a very complicated equation. We crack open the newest diet book and feel hopeful that *this* is the way up the mountain. This new plan will finally unstick us; we'll stop running in place. And then, of course, we'll be happy. And hot to boot!

> Statistically, the vast majority of diets are failures. The diet mentality can't compare to a long-term, holistic view of health.

People quickly gain back whatever weight they lost on a diet because they eventually return to their normal style of eating. Diets are simply too restrictive to be followed for the long term. And when we fall off the wagon, we tend to fall hard; in fact, studies show that 30–60 percent of dieters regain *more weight* than they lost on their diets. Everyone ends up feeling like a failure, pushed back into feeling half alive.

Diets also fail because they are incredibly superficial. You cannot diet or crash exercise your way to a healthy, balanced life. If you've tried to find balance in your life before and haven't met success, you know the space between unhealthy behaviors and healthy living is a deep river that sometimes runs cold and turbulent—it's not always easy to get across. Healthy living is truly about the emotional aspect of life as much as the physical side, and any plan that ignores this dimension is destined for failure in the long term.

Fortunately, this isn't *that* kind of diet book.

Let's not even call this a diet book at all—this is a holistic *healthy living guide*. The key word, perhaps, is *living*. Here is a plan that you can follow for life; it's not a short-term fix. You will be able to change your lifestyle so you can achieve your goals in all areas of your life while addressing your holistic self—your emotional and physical needs. This guide sets forth a plan for wholesome eating, fun exercise, and emotional exploration. No gimmicks, no restrictions.

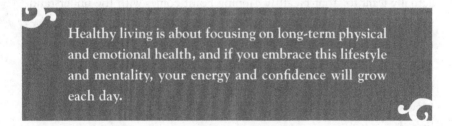

Healthy living is about focusing on long-term physical and emotional health, and if you embrace this lifestyle and mentality, your energy and confidence will grow each day.

I'm hereby establishing a guilt-free zone. You do not have to be perfect to be happy, healthy, or confident. It's difficult to make lifestyle changes, but it's even harder to do so when you waste valuable effort on berating yourself for "mistakes." So none of that here! Instead, we'll explore concepts like self-compassion and forgiveness.

This book is also not a one-size-fits-all approach. There are hundreds of ways to scale the mountain. If something in these pages really resonates and works for you—great. If not, that's fine, too. It doesn't mean you're a failure or lack willpower; it just confirms that your thought patterns, behaviors, and life situations are unique. These differences are exactly why, nestled within the chapters of this book, you'll find healthy living stories from dozens of inspiring women and men.

To reach your Healthy Tipping Point, you'll need to begin by consciously building momentum. At first, yes—you'll have to talk yourself into making healthy choices. If you've chosen to sit on the couch instead of exercising; if you've chosen to get takeout instead of cooking; if you've chosen to ruminate on all the things you want instead of the things you already have, you must change your behaviors. I promise that choosing the healthier option gets easier over time. And these choices add up to something amazing—your Healthy Tipping Point. This milestone occurs when the *true* definition of health—long-term emotional and physical wellness—finally clicks. You'll know you've hit your Healthy Tipping Point when you finally shift the focus from a short-term, appearance-based mind-set to long-term health and happiness pursuits. You begin to make the healthier choices not because you feel like you *have* to but because you actually *want* to. Your Healthy Tipping Point comes with the understanding that small efforts add up and that being healthy is not about perfection. This moment (or series of moments) occurs with an "aha!" realization that being healthy is not about gimmicks or restriction, and that getting healthy is a process that simply cannot happen in a vacuum. Health, food, fitness, happiness, love, work, family, friends, and life are all inextricably linked.

My story is not that unique. It's practically a cliché. But from it, I crafted a better, brighter future for myself.

My Healthy Tipping Point came when my best friend, Lauren, sat me down, looked me squarely in the eyes, and laid all my cards out on the table. She bluntly but lovingly told me I was making myself miserable.

My personal motto had been to "work hard, party hard," and I took both to the extreme, excelling in my class and hitting the bars hard three to five nights a week. I managed to keep my weight around an ideal number for four years of college by eating diet foods and occasionally skipping meals. A handful of times, I actually made it to the campus gym, usually motivated by guilt over something I had eaten the night before or by an impending spring break trip. Not once did I ever worry about the long-term physical damage my lifestyle inflicted on my body. But I did know that in the early morning, when all the fun was over, I felt unconfident, lazy, and unattractive.

Deep down, I knew something wasn't right about my behavior. I understood I was not living up to my full potential because of my late-night choices. But I did not know what to do to change my behavior. I didn't understand how to make healthier choices—or even what a "healthy choice" actually entailed. Every time I had tried to become "healthier" in the past, I sought out the lowest-calorie option without a glance at the ingredients list, shunned carbohydrates and desserts, and forced myself to go to the gym. To me, being "healthy" was synonymous with restriction. After a week of this punishing regimen, I would end up binge eating on cookies and then moan to my friends about my terrible lack of self-control.

Until I changed my definition of "health," being healthy was an all-or-nothing game that I inevitably lost.

It all clicked for me that fateful day my friend Lauren told it to me straight; yes, I was complaining constantly without taking any positive action, and yes, my behaviors were completely self-defeating. "I know you want more for yourself than this," Lauren said gently. And then she invited me on a run. "I think it would be good for you, not just physically, but mentally, too," she added.

Lauren said everything that a little voice inside of me had been whispering for so long. Vowing to be more proactive and forgiving toward myself, I decided that a run didn't seem like such a bad idea. Lauren was training for a marathon at the time, but she promised she would go slowly. "Heck,"

I thought, "I'll be fine." I honestly believed that I could bang out a few miles without trouble, but that was before I found myself staring at the sidewalk, hands on my knees and gasping for breath. Running was hard—really, really hard! And as I watched a little bead of sweat drip off my face and hit the blazing concrete, I had my Healthy Tipping Point. Just because it was hard didn't mean I should give up. Something within me lit on fire. I pulled myself straight and said, "Let's keep going—but I'm going to need to take walking breaks, too."

Perhaps no one was more surprised than me, but I stuck with it. Running had ignited something inside of me that I didn't even know existed— I had never been athletic in high school and certainly never exercised for any reason beyond feeling forced. But running—oh, running was different. For once, I exercised for fun and because I actually *wanted* to. That's not to say some runs weren't rough; of course I had bad runs. The bad runs were a blessing, though. They taught me to challenge myself, to push myself a little harder physically and mentally than I was used to doing. I grew more confident, and I felt less angry and depressed. Instead of running away from all my problems, I was tackling them head-on. I ran, literally, for my life.

Before my Healthy Tipping Point, I expended a great deal of energy focusing on eating, but not in a positive way. Many of my thoughts about food were negative. How many calories are in this? Can I eat this dessert if I skip the appetizer? What should I eat for breakfast tomorrow to make up for how much I'll drink tonight? Since my focus was always on the numbers—calories in, weight, grams of protein—I ended up having a very limited definition of why I ate what I ate. My food intake and behaviors were based on maintaining my shape, which allowed me to turn a blind eye to my other unhealthy behaviors, like eating tons of processed foods, drinking too much, and skipping out on regular exercise. Unfortunately, I now realize that far too many of us look at food, which is so essential and pleasurable, in such a negative light because we have been trained, in many ways, by our society to think this way.

With each mile I ran, my self-respect increased. Running taught me to see my body as a glorious and highly capable machine instead of just a vessel for decoration. Suddenly, function seemed more important than form. The more processed foods and alcohol I consumed, the worse I felt while running. My running was also negatively impacted by my irregular eating patterns. I decided to toss out all the odd "food rules" that I had picked up from years of chronic dieting and go back to the basics—I'd simply start eating *real food* in *regular portion sizes* at *regular intervals* throughout the day. After all, restricting and overeating processed foods made me feel terrible and did nothing for my energy levels.

In the past, I had read nutritional labels only to see how many calories were in a food, but I transitioned to looking further down the label, at the ingredients list. I'd jot down ingredients that I didn't recognize and Google them when I got home from the grocery store, horrified to discover that many ingredients I already knew were unhealthy lurked on ingredients lists under different names. I learned that trans fat, which has been shown to increase the risk of heart disease, was often listed as "partially hydrogenated oil" and that monosodium glutamate (MSG), a food additive loosely tied to a variety of chronic conditions, frequently lurked as "hydrolyzed vegetable protein." The more I looked into ingredient lists, the more aware I became that most people (myself included) were eating . . . junk. It was all *fake* food! Half of what I was consuming was created in a laboratory. So many of the food items that I thought were healthy prepackaged convenience foods were filled with artificial sweeteners, food colorings, additives, and flavor enhancers.

I began to replace diet foods with whole and natural foods. It sounds simple, but to me—it was revolutionary. Instead of yogurt packed with three different kinds of artificial sweeteners, sugary cereal, and sweetened dried cranberries for breakfast, I'd mix up a bowl of organic Greek yogurt, raw oats (trust me, raw oats really do taste amazing with yogurt!), and a sliced banana. Same general concept, but a cleaner ingredients list, more fiber and protein, less sugar, and an overall better nutritional profile. I began to understand that calories weren't the be-all and end-all, as I'd been led to be-lieve for so many years.

Eating wholesome foods satisfied me in a way that fake, processed foods couldn't. My energy skyrocketed. My digestion leveled out. My skin began to clear up. I slept better than ever before, and I woke up feeling rested and full of energy. I felt—and heck, *looked*—amazing. I shined from the inside out. For so many years, I had chalked up my depleted energy levels, head-aches, and stomach troubles to stress or genetics. I was shocked to realize how strongly and immediately better food choices affected my overall health. Food truly is a medicine (or poison) you take at least three times a day.

There was one problem with my new eating style—it simply wasn't as convenient as the processed foods, premade frozen dinners, and takeout that I had been living on. Our culture isn't geared toward real food; a quick jaunt around a shopping mall food court proves that it's often difficult to find fresh fruits, healthy vegetables, whole grains, or vegetarian protein sources. Instead of getting frustrated, I became proactive. I realized that peo-ple who ate clean, wholesome diets planned ahead—they went grocery shopping, packed healthy snacks, researched restaurants' menus online before deciding where to eat, and actually *cooked.*

And, yes—I had to learn to cook! I began my culinary journey by brows-ing fancy cookbooks, but I quickly got frustrated when I looked at the in-gredients list. "I don't have that in my pantry!" I'd think. "Where do you even find cocoa nibs in the grocery store?!" Or I'd go to the store, purchase all the strange ingredients for one meal, and realize that my home-cooked pad thai cost double what I'd pay at a restaurant.

After several months of burning rice on the bottom of my nice pots, I realized that healthy cooking isn't inherently complicated or time-consuming—it's all about how you approach it. I began to develop my own recipes with simple ingredients that most people have on hand. I also discovered many quick shortcuts that made cooking and preparing healthy foods so much easier. And best of all, I realized that healthy eating doesn't equal restriction; I could still enjoy my favorite foods and desserts after making some simple ingredient swaps. Don't worry—I won't keep my tricks a secret. You'll find many of my favorite recipes and cooking techniques throughout this book!

The exercise bug bit me, my sense of self-worth increased, and I'd learned my way around a kitchen. But the last piece of my Healthy Tipping Point puzzle fell into place when I discovered the world of healthy living blogs. The women and men behind these blogs shared real-life healthy living tips that I could actually apply to my life—not like those crazy fads that suggested I eliminate all white foods, like potatoes or pasta, or never eat after a certain time. Even more fantastic was the sense of community that these blogs fostered; reading the blogs each day felt like meeting up with friends for coffee. At the time, I had just moved to a new city and knew no one. Bloggers who didn't even know who I was understood and encouraged my new lifestyle choices.

In fact, I loved the blog world so much that I decided to join, too. I began the HealthyTippingPoint.com blog in June 2009 and have chronicled my life's adventures every day since. Blogging has kept me committed to being mentally and physically healthy—truly living—and shows me every single day that I'm not alone in the struggles I face. Throughout this book, you'll read dozens of inspiring stories from other bloggers and readers who underwent their own Healthy Tipping Point moment. Their stories illustrate a very important point: "healthy" looks different for different people. Although the core message is the same—move your body and eat real, wholesome foods—their experiences vary greatly. Healthy is about being strong and happy, not reaching a certain number on the scale. The individuals featured throughout this book have their own unique formula for and definition of success, and I hope their insights and experiences inspire you to be the best version of yourself, too.

> Health and happiness is a series of choices. Make one healthy choice today. Make another one tomorrow. Your efforts add up.

Through my journey, I've realized that healthy living is really about creating reverse inertia. Every choice you make—no matter how small—adds up, propelling you forward to the life you want to lead. Choosing to be mentally healthy encourages you to be physically healthy, and being proactive in your food and exercise choices boosts your self-esteem. Big changes don't happen overnight, but small choices occur in an instant. Make the choices for the life you want to lead.

To help you make these choices, this book is organized into the following three parts called "shifts"—not rules, not directions, not ultimatums. Instead, these shifts encourage simple changes in direction or attitude.

- "Get Real"
- "Eat Clean"
- "Embrace Strength"

While this book can certainly be read and enjoyed cover to cover, the idea behind its organization is that the advice in it can be applied slowly to your life, over several months or even a full year, which allows time to adjust to your new lifestyle choices. Slowly integrating the Healthy Tipping Point shifts will ensure you experience your own transformative Healthy Tipping Point moment (or moments!) and guarantee long-term success. Anyone who has crash dieted understands that fast, drastic results are rarely maintainable in the long run. Slow and steady wins the race, as the old saying goes.

My greatest hope is that, through this book, you will discover that you control your future and that you can choose to be as healthy and happy as possible. No restriction, no gimmicks, no denial required. Food can taste wonderful *and* fight aging, improve memory, boost fertility, and even increase happiness. Exercise can be a pleasant "me time" escape *and* help you achieve a toned, sexy shape. Neither food nor exercise has to be a source of strife or punishment, and you can come to peace with your amazing, wonderful body.

Health truly is about mental and physical balance, and I hope this holistic approach to true wellness helps propel you toward your best life. Trust me—no matter where you are on your journey, the view is worth the climb.

As you read through the book, you'll find fifty-two healthy choices—one for each week of the year, and one extra—that add up to something amazing.

1. Instead of simply changing the way you look, change the way you see. Positive changes begin in the mind.

2. Write down goals, obstacles, and rewards, and post the list in a highly visible location—like your bathroom mirror.

3. The first and last hour of the day set the tone for the rest of your life.

4. Drink water, a minimum of half your body weight in pounds in ounces of water. Chug at least another eight ounces for every fifteen minutes of exercise.

5. Stop buying into the Myth of the Someday. Proactively seek out happiness and acceptance *today*.

6. Don't let the media consume you—actively question and critique messages about beauty and attractiveness.

7. Lay the foundation for the life you want through your thoughts.

8. Ditch the Thin Ideal or the Muscular Ideal and focus on the Healthy Ideal, which looks different for different people.

9. Listen to your hunger cues—both physical and emotional—before making food choices.

10. When you feel negativity brewing, take a deep breath and choose to respond in a proactive, positive, and purposeful way.

11 Life isn't what happens *to* you. Life is what you *do* with the hand you're dealt.

12 Flip self-doubt around and use it as a powerful motivator.

13 You can't control everything that happens; however, you can change how you perceive and manage stress.

14 If you can't pronounce it, think twice about eating it.

15 If it comes in a box, bag, or wrapper, read the ingredients list.

16 Quick veggie fix: serve rice or pasta on a bed of raw baby spinach.

17 On Monday, bring five pieces of fresh fruit to work and store them in a basket on your desk. Snack on one every afternoon.

18 Give your brain time to catch up. In the middle of your meal, put your fork down for several minutes.

19 Keep cookies and baked goods in the freezer, not the pantry; you'll be less tempted to mindlessly munch.

20 Instead of counting calories, count servings of fruits and vegetables—aim for five to seven a day.

21 Fill half of your plate with plants.

22 To promote healthy digestion, drink a glass of water before eating breakfast, and wait to drink tea or coffee until after—not during—the meal.

23 Eat two tablespoons of ground flaxseed every day.

24 Body wash made from all-natural ingredients can be expensive. Dilute it with equal parts water to stretch your dollar.

25 Line produce drawers with organic paper towels; they'll absorb excess moisture and delay rot in fruits and vegetables. Replace the papers after every shopping trip.

26 Ditch the deli meat—make sandwiches with hummus, nut butter, or veggie burger patties.

27 Enjoy one "extra" when dining out—bread, appetizer, or dessert—not all three.

28 Instead of relying on pricey frozen dinners, make a healthy casserole on Sunday and freeze individual servings to enjoy throughout the week.

29 Create your own healthy nonstick spray by pouring olive oil into a clean food-grade spray bottle.

30 Scout online classified ads or garage sales to score high-quality appliances at a discount.

31 Make large batches of grains, like rice, ahead of time and freeze single-serving leftovers in an airtight container for up to three months. Reheat by warming in a skillet with a dash of water.

32 Don't exercise because you dislike your body. Exercise because you love your body.

33 Ditch the "all-or-nothing" mentality and begin by setting easily attainable fitness goals.

34 You cannot—and should not—do it all. When your personal or professional life is stressful, cut back on the intensity and duration of your workouts.

35 Lay out your workout gear the night before a morning workout. Bring your gym bag to work so you can tackle your evening workout right after you leave the office.

36 Exercise should add to, not detract from, your overall energy levels.

37 If you want to change your life, you must let go of fear. Failure is never trying.

38 Commit to taking a fifteen-minute walk at the same time of day, every day. This healthy habit adds up to 105 minutes of exercise each week!

39 When exercising outdoors, dress as if it is twenty degrees warmer.

40 Shop for athletic shoes late in the day—when your feet are naturally swollen—and buy a half a size to a size larger than your dress shoe size.

41 If you frequently travel for work, pack a workout DVD and exercise in your hotel room.

42 Swap motivating playlists with your workout buddy so you always have new, energizing tunes.

43 If you dread exercise, do an exercise experiment: commit to a different workout every week for two months. By trying eight different exercises, you're guaranteed to find something you enjoy.

44 Don't hide in the back—stand in the front the first time you attend a new class so you can easily see the instructor.

45 Rub a little spit in your goggles to prevent them from fogging up.

46 Every four to six weeks, "step back" your running by reducing overall mileage and intensity. This allows your body to heal and will ultimately make you a stronger, faster runner.

47 Collect sample workouts from fitness magazines and stash them in a folder. Whenever you feel stuck in a rut, pull out a sheet at random.

48 When using exercise equipment like an elliptical or a stair climber, vary the speed and resistance for a more effective workout.

49 Fold your yoga mat in half and then roll it up; this keeps the germy "outside" of the mat from touching the "inside."

50 Sign up for a race, like a 5K, to keep yourself accountable and committed to fitness.

51 A race is a celebration of your training. Training is a celebration of your body and spirit.

52 Training plans are guidelines, not absolutes. Listen to your body; don't blindly follow a plan.

53 Don't tackle speed and distance goals at the same time. Too much, too soon is a recipe for a training disaster.

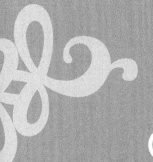

Part I

GET REAL

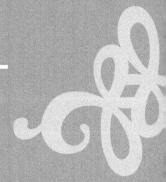

One

REFRAMING YOUR
HEALTH GOALS

The eyes are our bodies' most complex organ, second only to our brains. Composed of millions of tiny working parts, our eyes can focus on more than fifty objects in a single second. Humans are highly visual creatures, placing a premium on what we can see.

Every day, you're bombarded with images of what our society considers the ideal form. Whenever you casually turn the pages of a fashion magazine or flip through the channels on your television, your eyes soak up these images. And what we see is one definition of physical beauty. The desirable female shape is alarmingly thin, and attractive men are uniformly muscular, with broad shoulders and tapered waists. And regardless of whether you agree in your heart with the message behind this portrayal, your powerful eyes betray you, absorbing the high premium placed on appearance. In a glance, this message is transmitted to your brain. The idealized concept of beauty worms its way into your subconscious, and as a result, you may look at yourself in the mirror and sometimes feel defeated, unworthy, and broken in comparison.

Our society presents a very false and confusing ideal of beauty and often equates beauty and happiness with health. The vast majority of female models and celebrities are at a dangerously low and unhealthy weight and body mass index (BMI)—and, to add insult to injury, they are then Photoshopped to an unattainable level of thinness. Through photo-editing software, necks and legs are elongated, waists are shrunk, armpits almost disappear, cellulite is smoothed away, breasts are plumped, and pores fade away. Images of men are similarly deconstructed and manipulated. What's left is one humanly impossible representation of "beauty"—not health. The media's portrayal of the ideal female and male image is completely alien to the way real women and men look. We might as well be staring at images of creatures from another planet!

The primary message in our society is that our appearance is paramount. This outlook reinforces the following falsehoods:

- Your worth is based largely on your appearance.
- Eating is inherently restrictive or indulgent.
- Exercise is a form of punishment or repentance.
- Your happiness is tied closely to your appearance.
- Your looks are a direct reflection of how healthy you are on the inside, emotionally and physically.

Tackling healthy living from an appearance-based outlook is highly ineffective in the long run. This outlook encourages extreme and sudden lifestyle changes, like restricting certain foods or working out obsessively, which are impossible to maintain. If appearance-based goals are not immediately reached, people often feel discouraged and ashamed, which influences their ability to continue to make positive choices. Furthermore, the outlook has a severely limiting effect on a person's self-image; it's as if their entire life boils down to one pursuit: to look good. It's no wonder that, statistically speaking, most dieters (who are typically driven by appearance) regain all the weight they lost—plus a few pounds.

Now, no one is arguing that weight and health are unrelated. Carrying excess weight—or being underweight—can lead to a myriad of health problems, including an increased risk of heart disease and cancer. Maintaining a healthy weight, as well as a commitment to balanced eating and regular exercise, greatly reduces your susceptibility to acute and chronic diseases. And yet to boil down your Healthy Tipping Point journey to one thing—a number on the scale—is a great disservice to the complexity of the issue. Health and weight are related, but weight is not the final word on physical or emotional health. When we focus too much on weight, we often allow other very important health concerns to fall to the wayside: we rely on processed, chemically laden diet foods to lose weight; we restrict and then binge; we engage in negative self-talk and allow toxic relationships to form; we take up smoking to curb our appetite; we skip breakfast to "save calories"; we avoid lifting weights for fear of becoming bulky. A number on a scale does not tell the whole story on how healthy you are; the truth is that health looks different on different people. Health is not one size fits all. Health comes in a wide variety of body shapes, sizes, and—yes—weights.

Healthy Tipping Point Success Story: Laura, 25, Arizona

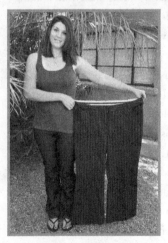

By the time I shuffled into the emergency room, I knew my situation was pretty bleak. I was terrified, my head was pounding, and I felt so weak. In a cold and sterile exam room, I nervously stepped on a scale, staring in horror. I was 320 pounds, my blood pressure was off the charts (300/200—the highest anyone at the hospital had ever seen in clinical practice), and I was only twenty-three years old.

Lying in the hospital bed, I felt so scared and defeated. With such high blood pressure, I was at risk for immediate stroke—or worse. As the doctors and nurses tinkered with my blood pressure medication, one nurse told me what no one else was willing to say out loud: I needed to lose weight and get healthy. As she talked, it dawned on me: I was literally killing myself. For the first time in my life, I was forced to accept the consequences of my bad lifestyle choices. And it was about much more than my blood pressure or being obese. It was clear to me that my choices were the direct result of my lack of self-worth or confidence.

I took a long, hard look at myself, and somewhere deep inside, I knew there was a girl who loved herself and wanted to live a healthy life. Right there and then, I decided to change. Not just for health reasons, but also because I knew I could change—and I wanted to.

As I drove home from the emergency room, I began to formulate a plan to get healthy—mentally and physically—the right way. To get physically healthy, I knew I had to change my eating and exercise habits immediately. I threw away all the junk food in the house. I went grocery shopping for the first time in a long time, and I bought healthy foods. With my doctor's approval, I started to walk every day. I went very slowly at first, but eventually, I worked up to three or four miles a day, several times a week. After I had lost more than one hundred pounds, I joined a gym and tried lots of fun classes, like BodyPump and spinning. I eventually transitioned from walking to running, too. I even ran a half-marathon!

I quickly realized that I also needed to work on my relationship with myself, as well as my relationships with other people. For too long, I had put other people's happiness above my own. You don't get to be 320 pounds by putting yourself first. I learned to deal with the emotional triggers that caused me to eat out of emotion, and I developed healthier coping mechanisms, like exercise. It took a while to transform my thinking, and I still struggle with confidence issues from time to time, but I began to understand that I could create the life I wanted. I ended up going back to school so I could finish college. I got a job in a field that makes me feel fulfilled. And just a few weeks after my transformative trip to the emergency room, I met a wonderful man who loves me regardless of the number of the scale. He loved me when I was over 300 pounds, and he loves me now.

In total, I've lost 139 pounds. I'm six feet tall, and while I'll never be petite and thin, I like my curvy body just fine. Healthy comes in many different sizes, and it's about so much more than your weight. It's about who you are on the inside, too. There are no tricks or shortcuts to physical and mental health—you just have to work hard and love yourself. This journey allowed me to rediscover who I am—and I love what I've gained.

> Instead of simply changing the way you look, change the way you see. Positive changes begin in the mind.

First things first—you must begin your Healthy Tipping Point journey with the right attitude about *why* you want to make healthier choices. And the right attitude means adopting a health-centered mind-set, not an appearance-based outlook.

Approaching life with a health-centered mind-set is freeing because it removes an unnecessary pressure to reach a certain number on the scale or fit into a particular pant size. It takes the focus off the short term and places it firmly where it should be: the duration of your long, happy life. It's easier to make healthy choices while focusing on your long-term health, since there is more room for moderation and balance in food and exercise choices. And, perhaps most important, a health-centered mind-set is holistic, addressing not only your physical health needs, but also your emotional needs.

Ironically, developing a health-centered mind-set will actually do more for your looks than an appearance-based outlook. When you strive to be physically and mentally healthy, you glow from the inside out. Health is apparent in your bright skin, strong nails, strong hair, firmer body, and clear eyes. Health is beautiful, in all of its many shapes and sizes.

So, let's get our health-centered mind-set in focus:

- Eat a diet filled with natural, minimally processed foods and enjoy treats, fast food, or other processed foods in moderation.
- Make dietary choices that leave you feeling nourished and energized.
- Regularly exercise to improve cardiovascular health, promote bone density, and maintain a healthy weight.
- Respect the only body you'll ever have by drinking in moderation, reducing unnecessary stressors, not smoking, engaging in safe sex, getting enough sleep, and drinking enough water.
- Carve out personal time to relax or enjoy a hobby in your day-to-day life.
- Cultivate a strong sense of self-worth.
- Internalize the message that our society's idealized version of beauty has *nothing* to do with health.

Specific ways to develop and implement these healthy habits are described throughout this book. You'll also be able to draw inspiration from the Healthy Tipping Point success stories, which include experiences and ideas from people who have successfully implemented health-centered thinking in their own lives. Just as health looks different for different people, the approach to healthy living varies from person to person. Maybe some of these insights will resonate with you, too.

Healthy Tipping Point Success Story:
Ryan, 29, Utah

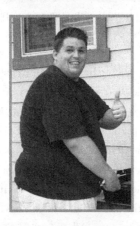 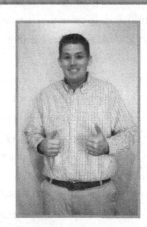

I was overweight as a child, and my parents were overweight, too. I packed on the pounds through college and during the beginning of my career, and by July 2009, I weighed about 400 pounds. I tried a lot of different weight-loss programs, and I even had success with a few of them. But my problem wasn't losing weight; it was losing weight without gaining it back.

My approach in the past has always been to justify my behavior. I would think, "One cookie isn't going to hurt," or "I already exercised twice this week; that's two more times than I usually do." I would blow off my goals because I was never really serious about my health. Basically, I wanted to lose weight without having to really change. The hard truth is that there's no quick fix. The problem was really my mental approach to weight loss. I had to find a *reason* to change, even when the change was hard.

One day, I rushed to the doctor's complaining of shoulder pain, and he pulled out an EKG machine right away. My blood pressure wasn't extremely high (140/82), but the doctor was sure that because of my size, my left arm pain indicated that I was having a heart attack. . . . Turns out that it was just a sprain.

After several other experiences where my weight was an issue—like avoiding stairs and having trouble with my golf swing—something clicked in my brain. I want to grow old with my wife. I want my boys to have wrestling matches with their dad. I want to be healthy for my family. Like a flash, all of the other experiences leading up to that moment played back in my head. I told myself then that I *would* change—my trigger was pulled. I haven't looked back, but I remember these events every day. They drive me and keep me motivated.

With two young boys and a desk job, making healthy living a part of my life was a challenge. The only way I could do it was to wake up ridiculously early (4:30 a.m.!) and get my workout done before the kids got up. Making sure I had time to exercise was very important because it is a huge stress reliever. Of course, it was hard sometimes, but all I had to do was remind myself that I wasn't just exercising for myself—it was for my family, too.

If there's one thing I would recommend to people looking to improve their lives, it is to find your trigger. Find the one thing that switches on your focus, and make your new way of life a priority. When you're struggling, remember your trigger and use it for your last burst of strength. At the end of the day, it's simply mind over matter. You have to decide you want to change. And then you will.

Let's Get Going!

In addition to a focus on health over appearance, the most important precursor to experiencing a Healthy Tipping Point transformation is motivation. It is the matchstick and the wood, the catalyst required to ignite the fire and keep it burning. The trouble with motivation is that most of us focus only on the *initial* motivation to change, not putting much thought into creating a long-term self-support system. And when we focus on short-term success, it is relatively easy to be derailed when confronted with an obstacle ("I might as well give up now!") or even a small success ("I've earned the right to slack off").

To experience a true, lasting Healthy Tipping Point that stays on course despite daily challenges, you must first change how you approach getting—and staying—motivated.

Just as a tiny amount of friction causes a matchstick to ignite into a small flame, Matchstick Motivation (short-term motivation) is relatively easy to come by. Maybe your pants are too tight, you've picked up that pack of cigarettes again, or you went an entire weekend without eating a single vegetable. And suddenly, you're feeling super motivated to change. Perhaps you even bought this book after a Matchstick Motivation moment! How many Mondays have you woken up and vowed that you'll *never* slack off during the weekends again, that *this* is the week you change your life? The trouble with Matchstick Motivation is that it only creates a small, intense flame of desire to change—and this flame tends to burn out quickly because of the strong connection between Matchstick Motivation moments and appearance-based thinking.

Matchstick Motivation is also troublesome because of the restrictive and unmaintainable methods most people use to reach their desired life changes. Pants too tight? Time to crash diet! No veggies? Better go on that detox! Figuring out why these extreme methods usually fail will help you understand how to create real and lasting motivation.

- **Guilt Tripping:** Guilt is the ultimate Matchstick Motivation emotion. We pitch our desired life changes to ourselves, the language dripping in hurt and shame. "Why can't you just put down that cookie, you cow?" or "No one will ever love if you don't quit smoking those cancer sticks." In terms of healthy living, people often return to this technique over and over again because it is quite effective in the short term.

  One big problem with guilt is that it promotes fear-based decision making. Instead of focusing on your growth and potential, guilt tripping ultimately makes your dreams smaller and more confined because you're focusing on what you cannot do, not what you *want* to do. Second, guilt is ineffective in the long term because it ties healthy choices to punishment. Subconsciously, guilt links healthy eating and exercise—two very positive actions—with deeply negative emotions. This makes it very difficult to stay on task in the long term.

- **Perfectionism:** Another common type of Matchstick Motivation is perfectionism. It's a solemn vow that, from this point forward, you will be flawless in your food choices and exercise habits. At first, perfectionism can seem quite relieving, especially on the heels of several poor decisions. The very absolute nature of perfectionism can be soothing and reduce anxiety because it offers the promise that you'll never screw up again. Buoyed by this promise, it's easy to make healthier choices for the first few days or weeks, with each impeccable choice reaffirming your commitment to perfection.

  Perfect, of course, simply doesn't exist. This Matchstick Motivation is usually corrupted the first time you "screw up" by missing a gym date or eating something outside of your strict diet. These screwups, of course, aren't really mistakes at all, but simply part of being a human being with a busy schedule and many competing responsibilities. People who embrace the extreme of perfectionism in healthy living often wildly swing back to utter abandon, falling off the wagon far and hard. After all, the perfectionist will reason, if you're not doing it perfectly, what's the point of doing it at all? Perfectionism is so dangerous precisely because it endorses this highly limited, obsessive type of thinking, which can beget a host of emotional and physical disorders.

- **External Motivation:** Feeling weak-willed, some people will appeal to outsiders to inflict external motivation on their psyche. Utilizing external motivation, such as the feedback from a critical lover or a toxic relative, may drive the person to go through the motions of healthy eating and exercise. Alternatively, we may try to prove the external motivator wrong under the guise of "I'll show them!" On a larger sociological scale, we often compare ourselves to our society's strict—and unattainably Photoshopped—definition of beauty and sex appeal as motivation to succeed.

Submitting to an external motivator can also cause us to self-sabotage when we tire of the control. And last, external, negative motivation fails because it cannot produce the same type of commitment that comes from self-created, positive motivation.

- **Bribery:** The final method of enacting Matchstick Motivation is classic bribery. Unable to drum up internal motivation without a reward system, we may use bribery as a way to encourage ourselves to stick to healthy choices. For example, many diets promote a "free day" during which dieters can eat anything they want, provided they stick to the plan for the rest of the week.

  No one can argue that bribery isn't effective. There is a time and a place for bribery and rewards. I can't deny the allure of a back massage after a hard workout or a mindless evening in front of the television after a busy workday! However, small rewards can begin to lose their appeal over time, forcing you to always up the ante. If you become overly reliant on bribery, it can be difficult to get focused without the promise of a metaphorical carrot. And using food as a reward for healthy eating and exercise can be dangerous, since it defines food in very limited terms—some as healthy but undesirable and other foods as unhealthy but special. Plus, one *really* "off" day can actually unravel a whole week's worth of work. It's usually healthier—mentally and physically—to spread out smaller desserts and proper servings of salty snacks through the week instead of jamming your body full of junk food on your "free" day.

Because these Matchstick Motivation methods—guilt tripping, perfectionism, external motivation, or bribery—often result in short-term results, we tend to return to these methods to better ourselves. However, these methods end up doing more harm than good, the quintessential one step

forward, two steps back. Human nature guarantees that short-term motivation will fall to the wayside when confronted with life's many ups and downs.
Expecting a negative, short-term motivator to result in positive, long-term
changes is ridiculous.

FLIP YOUR NEGATIVITY

Positive thinking is a self-fulfilling prophecy. To paraphrase Henry Ford,
whether you think you can or think you can't, you're probably right. To
reduce or eliminate negative thinking in all areas of your life, you must first
consciously acknowledge that you're doing it in the first place! Many of us
let negativity flitter in and out of our thoughts and words without realizing
the subconscious damage such feelings inflict. Alternatively, we might not
even "hear" our negative thoughts but instead feel negative emotions, such
as sadness, being overwhelmed, anxiety, grief, or nervousness.

Once you've acknowledged the negative thought or emotion, replace it
with a positive but realistic thought. Studies show that positive thinking is
most effective when it's believable. If you constantly experience the same
negative thoughts, it can be helpful to identify a positive antidote in advance, as listed below. Positive thinking is also more effective if it is specific. Covering up strong negative emotions with a trite statement such as,
"There's always a silver lining," might not make you feel any better. Instead,
consciously list the silver linings. Make yourself focus on the good instead
of the bad, and soon your mood and motivation will grow exponentially.

NEGATIVE THOUGHT	POSITIVE THOUGHT
I'm a failure.	Making mistakes is human, and I'm going to do the best I can.
I'm so ugly.	Beauty comes from the inside out, and I have many great qualities, such as . . .

I will never be able to . . .	I will create a plan, act on my goals, and I'm not going to give up.
I'm so shy; people are going to judge me.	Most people are nervous in groups; just concentrate on being friendly to a few people.
I have no energy and feel so useless.	I'm going to put in some work (five minutes, an hour, any reasonable time) and see how I feel then.
I can't do this; I'm not good enough.	I don't need to be perfect; I just need to work hard and put in the effort.
Life is horrible—so many problems!	This life is what I make of it; I can only control my reactions to events.
I'll never have everything I want.	Here is a list of the intangible things I have. . . .
I don't have the willpower to change.	It's never too late to change, and I'm going to take things one step at a time.

As Albert Einstein famously said, doing the same thing over and over again and expecting different results is the definition of insanity. If you want to truly change your behavior, you have to change your motivational methods. By approaching life changes in a Healthy Tipping Point fashion, you can create a type of motivation that grows and multiplies with each success, thereby ensuring commitment over the long term. Just as fire requires oxygen to burn, lasting motivation feeds on a well-planned and proactive lifestyle shift that focuses on the long term *in addition to* the short term.

Remember Laura's Matchstick Motivation moment when she was rushed to the emergency room with alarmingly high blood pressure? She turned that moment into a lifestyle change by adopting a positive and proactive mind-set. These two components—being positive and proactive—stand in sharp contrast to the negative Matchstick Motivation methods described earlier and are key for long-term success.

Real motivation is not just an innate ability, available only to the few lucky people born with the gene. It's a skill you can teach yourself. First, you need to consciously practice the methods for real motivation; eventually, these habits will become intuitive, and you'll be filled with lasting motivation to succeed in your healthy living goals.

Here is the formula for long-term motivation.

Grace + Appreciation + Focus = Long-Term Motivation

The first thing to notice about this magical formula is that each component is a *positive* action. The overarching reason why most people fail to drum up long-term motivation is that they approach motivation in a negative fashion, either by guilt, bribery, or comparing themselves to others. To experience a Healthy Tipping Point transformation, you must begin to approach life changes in terms of what you *can* do and *will* do.

- **Grace:** It is very easy to be positive when you're doing things correctly, but most of us slip into negative self-talk the moment we mess up. To circumvent this negative self-talk, try incorporating grace into your thought patterns and instituting a policy of forgiveness for mistakes, both past and current. Popular diet advice usually focuses on being "perfect," leaving very little room for day-to-day balance. Such rigid thinking is bound to end in disappointment, and without the supportive safety net of grace, many end up throwing in the towel altogether—"If I cannot be perfect, why even try?" On the other hand, grace encourages us to bounce back and try again. Learning to let things go so we can try on another day is essential to living a healthy lifestyle, day by day.

Grace is not a hall pass to constantly screw up, mindlessly absolve ourselves, and screw up again. Quite the opposite—grace requires that you take a good, hard look at your behavior and implement changes based on your findings. Following this period of introspection, you let the mistake go. When we fall off the healthy living bandwagon and focus too strongly on our errors, we engage in self-sabotaging behavior, such as restriction, negative talk, or compulsive exercise, as atonement.

- **Appreciation**: Most of us find it extremely awkward to engage in self-appreciation. But it is an absolute must if you're seeking out long-term motivation. Appreciate what you have done in the past (however small!) and celebrate each positive choice you are making in the present. By focusing on your accomplishments and abilities, you reinforce the Healthy Tipping Point belief that small decisions can add up to something amazing.

Beyond reminding yourself of your positive actions, it can also be helpful to practice appreciation for your body at its most basic level: as a vessel for your spirit. For example, flip negative connotations about exercise ("I'm so slow! This is too hard! Everyone is staring at me!") by celebrating sweat as a form of appreciation for your body ("I am lucky to be able to walk. My body is getting stronger every day"). Especially when combined with grace, appreciation can help you move past any highly destructive perfectionist thoughts.

Furthermore, adopting a positive mind-set, especially in the face of obstacles, actually makes you work harder.[1] In a recent psychological study, participants who were asked to make optimistic predictions about how long it would take to finish a stressful task spent more time working on the task—and were thus more successful in achieving their goals—than people who were asked to make realistic predictions. Give yourself some credit—you can and will succeed. You just have to believe it's possible.

- **Focus:** One reason why Matchstick Motivation moments are so ineffective is that these knee-jerk reactions, usually in response to negative emotions or experiences, don't come with a solid, realistic plan. Thus, the third part of our long-term motivation equation is that you must plan for success.

Planning for Success

Grace and appreciation go a long way to cultivating a positive attitude toward healthy living, which is paramount for success, but good intentions without a well-developed plan are meaningless. Basically, if you don't buckle down and focus, you're going to blow it. People may believe they have developed a plan by simply stating a goal—"I want to become fitter" or "I want to be skinnier"; however, such loosely defined goals actually set us up for failure because these goals lack focus.

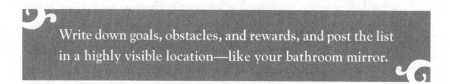

Write down goals, obstacles, and rewards, and post the list in a highly visible location—like your bathroom mirror.

The first step to developing focus is to create a detailed Healthy Tipping Point plan that includes the following:

- Short-term and long-term emotional and physical goals, with a focus on health-based goals (not appearance-based goals)
- A list of why your goals are important

- Step-by-step plans to achieve the short-term and long-term goals
- Clearly defined terms of success
- A summary of potential obstacles and solutions
- An outline of milestone markers (rewards)

Just as guilt and bribery can be negative motivators for all areas of your life, not just healthy living, the Healthy Tipping Point plan for long-term motivation can also be applied to your personal, professional, and spiritual life. In fact, your healthy living goals might intersect and influence your other goals (and vice versa); for example, one of your healthy living long-term goals might be to achieve a healthy body-fat percentage, and your personal goal might be to conceive without the aid of fertility drugs. Furthermore, it's important to consider the whole picture and not set goals for each area of your life in a vacuum. Perhaps your healthy living goal is to exercise five days a week, but your professional goals require that you work sixty-hour weeks. Achieving both of these goals fully might not be possible—and that's totally okay. Setting yourself up to fail is the worst thing you can do! Set yourself up to succeed instead.

To determine your short-term and long-term healthy living goals, begin by asking yourself the Big Question: *What do I want out of my life, and how does healthy living fit in?*

The Big Question can be quite nerve-wracking if you're not exactly sure what you want out of your life; if you're stuck, focus instead on defining your desired emotional state, not a list of achievements or material possessions. Perhaps you seek adventure; maybe you just want to experience contentment. Do you want to feel strong and confident? Do you want to find balance and peace? Do you want to improve your health and be more active for your family? Do you want to stop obsessive thoughts when it comes to food and exercise, or do you wish you could motivate yourself to care a little bit more? Once you've begun to define the answer to the Big Question, you can begin to create a list of short-term and long-term goals that will help move you toward your desired state.

FLUSH WITH HAPPINESS

Think money is the answer to all your problems? One study of twenty-two lottery winners determined that the joys of winning wads of cash wore off after just a few months, and afterward, the winners were not significantly happier than a control group. Feeling successful—*not* being rich—is most closely tied to happiness. If you want to make yourself happier, set attainable goals relating to your health, personal life, and career, and develop a plan to meet them.

Imagine your answer to the Big Question as the top of a pyramid. Directly below are your long-term goals, which may be related to a variety of areas in your life: personal, spiritual, and professional. Short-term goals lay the foundation for achieving your long-term goals. If your long-term healthy living goal is to run a marathon, short-term goals that will help you achieve this goal may include running a 5K, a 10K, and a half-marathon.

Goals are most effective when they are stated clearly, quantifiable, and include a deadline. The long-term goals of "I want to become fitter" and "I want to be skinnier" can be transformed into "By next summer, I want to be able to do biceps curls with thirty-pound weights and run a ten-minute mile," and "Over the next year, I'd like to lose enough weight to fall within the healthy weight range for my height."

Additionally, enumerate why each of your goals is important. If you cannot think of why a goal is truly important to you or the reasons seem superficial, it might be necessary to reframe your goal in terms that fit in with your answer to the Big Question. We often get hung up on an appearance-based outlook, fixating on achieving an arbitrary "goal weight," and fail to focus on what *really* matters to us—health, love, happiness, adventure. Take the time to consider what achieving these goals will mean to you and how you hope the experiences will enrich your life.

By laying out your short- and long-term goals, you create a step-by-step plan for success. Smaller, well-defined milestones aid in motivation and boost positive thinking, since your long-term goals seem more realistic and attainable.

Another important component of your Healthy Tipping Point plan is to identify any potential obstacles that may arise as you pursue your short- and long-term goals. Common obstacles may include hitting a plateau when weight loss or fitness gains stall out; becoming overwhelmed with family or work obligations; or suffering an injury or sickness. By identifying obstacles and crafting solutions in advance, you'll be better equipped to handle setbacks. After all, the reality is that success is not linear—healthy living is a balancing act. With a little planning, grace, and appreciation, you'll be able to bounce back and prevent small bumps from completely derailing you.

Examples of ways to overcome common obstacles include:

- If work becomes so busy that it is impossible to cook healthy meals during the week, reserve Sunday afternoon to precook and freeze several healthy dishes.
- If you suffer a lower body injury during training for a half-marathon, take up a nonimpact exercise alternative, such as swimming, and plan to run another race once you've healed.
- If you continue to suffer from appearance-based anxiety, schedule an appointment with a therapist to discuss ways to boost your self-esteem.

The final key to staying on track and motivated is milestone markers, which are essentially rewards to celebrate your achievements. Ideally, your rewards should reinforce positive behaviors, not oppose them, which keep the rewards from turning into negative bribes. Examples of reinforcing rewards for health-centered goals include:

- Purchasing new workout clothes or gear
- Adding new workout songs to your playlist

- Scheduling a back massage or other spa treatment
- Organizing a "hike date" with friends
- Hosting a healthy dinner party

Many experts say that it can be dangerous to tie rewards to food, because it casts food into two restrictive lights: "good for me but undesirable" and "bad for me but desirable." That's the trouble with "splurge days," a concept that is very popular in many diet books. On a splurge day, you can eat anything you want (be "bad") because you were "good" all week. The splurge day concept can create a dangerous dichotomy in your mind. If you feel very emotional toward food or unsure of your ability to stay on track with healthy eating habits, keep your attitude about eating as positive as possible by not tying rewards to food. You can still have "discretionary foods" every day (more about discretionary foods on page 119), but consider your favorite fried food or sweet treat as *part* of your balanced diet, not a delicious exception to it.

Now—this Healthy Tipping Point plan for long-term success is not a metaphorical plan. It is a tangible document. It is very, very important to actually write (or type) out your goals, reasons, obstacles, and rewards. Stick the list in a highly visible location (on the refrigerator or your bathroom mirror is a good place) and cross off items as you go. Alternatively, your plan could be written in your diary or your blog. The most important thing is that you take the time (writing out a lifestyle plan should take *at least* ten minutes!) to cement your goals in your head and heart.

It is extremely easy to forget your accomplishments . . . and yet so hard to let go of your shortcomings. Checking off successes will boost your confidence and remind you how far you've come. Your Healthy Tipping Point plan will become a source of inspiration and motivation—proof that you can, and will continue to, succeed.

Healthy Tipping Point Success Story:
Donielle, 37, California

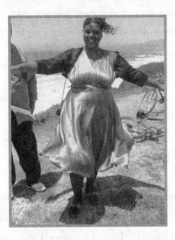

My health struggle is recurrent pregnancy loss—I've had three miscarriages. My normally optimistic spirit, which stayed largely intact after miscarriages one and two, started to nosedive after the third. I researched RPL for hours on end, read medical journal articles, made complicated to-do lists, and got ready to knock on doctors' doors to find a cure. However, amidst all that action, I only became more and more depressed. I realized that I needed a way to cope "in the now." I had been implicitly telling myself, "I'll be happy when the baby is finally here," which was another way of saying, "I'll be miserable until a baby is finally here."

I read *On Fertile Ground: Healing Infertility* by Helen Adrienne, and the book changed my life. Among many wonderful insights, Helen writes a lot about identifying the strengths that come out of any adversity. At first, like Helen predicts, I hated the idea—I certainly didn't see any blessings in RPL, and it made me slightly annoyed to even consider that there could be something good about RPL. The whole experience of repeated miscarriages just felt so unfair; it was proof of a cruel universe.

Yet as I read more, I realized that it has been because of infertility that I took the first real, effective, and consistent steps toward being healthier. I had gradually gained sixty pounds during the last decade, but now I am improving my diet and developing a consistent workout routine. So far, I've lost twenty-five pounds.

Infertility gave me the motivation I needed to change my life. Nothing before has worked for long-term motivation—not vanity, not common sense, not even a high blood sugar reading! I always just said, "I'll improve my health someday," and someday never came. Until now.

After years of poor health habits, what are the odds that I would have refocused effectively on how I eat and move if my pregnancy journey had been simple and quick? I would likely have gotten caught up in caring for my baby and continued to stall in my commitment to becoming healthy. Who knows where I'd be today?

The Healthy Tipping Point Hours

The Healthy Tipping Point philosophy is about small choices. These efforts build on one another, ultimately having a tremendously positive impact on your emotional and physical health. When healthy living is viewed in terms of small efforts and not sweeping, dramatic changes, a lifestyle change seems much more manageable.

There are two hours of your day that greatly impact the emotional and physical tone of the rest of your life. These hours are known as the Healthy Tipping Point hours. To achieve short- and long-term goal success, you must carve out room to grow and thrive, both in body and in spirit, during these important hours.

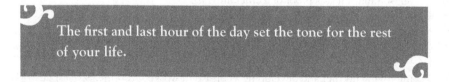

The first and last hour of the day set the tone for the rest of your life.

Changing the way you behave during the Healthy Tipping Point hours can be completely transformative. The first hour is about being emotionally and physically proactive, while the last hour is about winding down. Both hours, while so different, have a profound impact on your attitude, healthy, relationships, and even your work.

THE POWER HOUR

I'm nicknaming the first hour the Power Hour because this pivotal first hour influences the entire day. If you want to have a healthy, happy, productive day, you'd better be healthy, happy, and productive during the Power Hour. Does this mean we should leap out of bed and spring into immediate action the moment the alarm clock rings? Nope! In fact, this sudden, stressful jolt is the exact opposite of what we should do during the Power Hour. This critical hour isn't about work—it's about taking care of *you*.

Let's develop a Power Hour ritual that leaves you feeling organized, refreshed, and renewed. Most of us already have some type of morning routine that revolves around showering, eating, checking e-mails, getting our children ready for school, and other mundane tasks. A Power Hour ritual is a little more focused and purposeful.

A Power Hour ritual involves several components in addition to your normal morning tasks of getting ready and getting out the door. It's probably necessary to set your alarm clock a little bit earlier to give yourself the space to do these Power Hour activities. I promise—it's worth it.

1. **Attitude Influence:** At the moment you wake up, you are somewhere between sleep and alertness, between subconsciousness and consciousness. At this juncture, you are your most creative and relaxed. In fact, you may have noticed that you have your best ideas after a good night's sleep. Maybe you wake up with solutions to vexing problems or feel more emotionally resolved. This is because your mind is the most *open* during the first moments of the Power Hour.

    Your mind's openness means you are very vulnerable to attitude influence during these waking moments. The old adage "getting up on the wrong side of the bed" rings true. If you wake up in a nasty mood, this attitude will influence your entire day. If you happen to wake up in a positive state, you might declare, "I have a really good feeling about today!" for no reason other than you were happy during the first few moments of the Power Hour.

The moment you turn off the alarm clock, engage in attitude influence by breathing deeply and focusing your thoughts on having a happy, healthy day. Don't even get out of bed. Allow your body and mind to ease into the day in a slow, gentle way, as you would guide a baby into a warm bath. Try repeating a positive mantra—such as, "Today will be a good day," "I will honor my body today," or "I will embrace and enjoy life in a balanced way." If you struggle with anxiety or depression, it is especially helpful to pause for a moment of gratitude. Enumerating blessings—especially ones we often take for granted (food, safety, house, health)—adjusts your attitude to be grateful, positive, and proactive. Breathing deeply during this short, five-minute meditative session will oxygenate your brain and muscles, further preparing you for the day.

The key to successfully influencing your attitude is to not let the stressors of everyday life creep into your mind during these first waking moments. Try not to ruminate over your upcoming workday or the chores you must complete. Instead, allow yourself to focus on goodness and deep, steady breathing.

2. **Stretching:** Stretching during the Power Hour continues to ease you, physically and mentally, into the day. It warms up your joints and increases blood flow while simultaneously awakening your mind. Many people find that practicing yoga during Power Hour elevates their mood and sets positive intentions for the rest of the day; however, not everyone can dedicate time to the mat first thing in the morning (and personally, I struggle to feel very Zen first thing in the morning). Fortunately, stretching during the Power Hour does not need to be time-consuming.

Stretch at the same time you engage in attitude influence. Reach your arms over your head, flex your feet, arch your back, and sit up in bed and reach for your toes, all while repeating your positive morning mantras. Alternatively, stretch during your shower (a warm shower will relax your muscles as you stretch) or while you complete other morning tasks, like cooking breakfast, playing with your children, or walking the dog.

3. **Hydrate First:** More than 50 percent of Americans drink coffee as part of their morning ritual—and most of us java lovers drink three to four cups every day.[2] Before slamming back a cup of coffee or eating breakfast, be sure to drink a large glass of water. Water is the basis for all of our biological functions, and coffee is inherently dehydrating. Drinking water within the Power Hour will increase your alertness and improve digestion. And, of course, staying hydrated is an extremely important part of being healthy, so you should continue to drink water all day long.

   The jury is still out on coffee consumption. Some studies say that coffee can be part of a healthy diet—fighting heart disease, diabetes, and even Parkinson's disease—while others argue it increases hypertension and accelerates bone loss. And while many java lovers adore the caffeine boost, too much can result in frayed nerves and digestive issues. The devil may be in dosage, not just on a daily basis but in the long term, too. Two cups a day might not sound like a lot, but that's fourteen cups a week and nearly 730 cups a year. If you overload your coffee with creamer or sugar, the caloric impact adds up, too.

   Coffee is delicious and, for many busy people, is the fuel that gets them through a busy day. Starting the Power Hour off with water will

Drink water, a minimum of half your body weight in pounds in ounces of water. Chug at least another eight ounces for every fifteen minutes of exercise.

energize you, too, but it's the type of energy that begets more energy. Coffee, on the other hand, always ends in a caffeine-withdrawal crash . . . unless you drink more of it.

If you don't want to give up your beloved java, that's fine—just don't make it the first drink of the day. Wait to drink coffee until after your day has already begun; you may find that once you get going, you don't need the coffee as badly as you thought you did.

If you're a multiple-cup drinker, try drinking one cup of coffee *after* the Power Hour and then switching to tea. You can also try drinking coffee one morning and just tea the next, alternating between the two to reduce your overall coffee consumption. Packed with antioxidants, tea isn't as harsh on your digestive system as coffee and can contain considerably less caffeine. Drinking tea to get over a coffee addiction is kind of like wearing a nicotine patch—it will help you slowly reduce consumption without triggering withdrawal symptoms, like a headache. Eventually, you may be able to switch to a healthier tea (like green tea) or just wholesome, simple water.

4. **Healthy Fuel:** After drinking water, the fourth component of the Power Hour is to feed your body healthy fuel. Starting your day off with a balanced, stabilizing breakfast has both mental and physical ramifications. Healthy eating is explored in-depth in the "Eat Clean" section of this book.

5. **The Top Three:** Last, but certainly not least, take a few moments during the Power Hour to identify your top three goals for the day. These "microgoals" may be personal, professional, and/or health related. Too often our days slip by under a crush of tedious menial tasks. You must set the intention to tackle larger, more important goals, such as exercising, finishing an important document at work, or preparing a healthy dinner for your family. Your top three can be scribbled on a scrap piece of paper, written in your date book, entered in your calendar, or e-mailed to yourself.

Most workers come in, sit at their desks, and get lost for a significant amount of time checking e-mails or browsing online. You may find that you are more productive overall if you tackle one of the top three items immediately after the Power Hour. Don't leave your priorities to the last minute!

The top three can also be identified the night before, during the second Healthy Tipping Point hour, known as the Restorative Hour. If you find it is difficult to mentally switch from daytime responsibilities to rest, writing the top three before bed can help put your mind at ease.

The Restorative Hour

Make the last hour of the day your Restorative Hour. Sounds nice, doesn't it? Oh yes, we could all use some restoring after a busy day. But most of us don't carve out that time. We either go-go-go until we simply face-plant in bed or we surf the Internet until our eyelids become heavy. If you're like me, you're prone to mindlessly zoning out in front of the television!

Just as we need to take a few minutes during the Power Hour to ease into the morning, we need time to relax and eventually ease into sleep during the Restorative Hour. Developing a Restorative Hour ritual decreases stress, improves your sleep, and moves you closer to your larger goals.

1. **Tidy Up:** An hour before bed, take fifteen minutes to tidy up your house. Do the dishes, wipe down the countertops, put away the kids' jackets, and take out the dog. These tasks will prepare you to have a better tomorrow. When you wake up, your house will be organized and pleasant.
2. **Eat Something Small:** Many diet books suggest not eating after a certain hour, claiming eating too late will cause you to gain weight. This recommendation is far too simplified. You will not gain weight, no matter when you eat, as long as you are not overeating throughout the day as a whole. However, it's not healthy to eat a

huge meal right before lying down; your body will spend too much energy on digestion when it should be resting and recovering. Aim to eat dinner several hours before the Restorative Hour. If you're hungry during the last hour of the day, eat a small, healthy snack.

3. **Let Go of Stressors:** Let's say you had a meeting with your boss that went terribly, and now you can't stop thinking about all the work you need to do, even though it's 9:45 at night. After tidying up, sit down on the couch and make a short list of errands or tasks to tackle the next day. This list making may replace writing the top three in the morning, or you may use the time at night to write down more trivial chores that nag at your brain—"Buy toilet paper" or "Call about the electric bill." Once you've got all your anxiety-producing thoughts on paper, allow yourself to relax. Now that they have been written down, you won't forget to do the tasks.

4. **Turn Off Electronics:** Many of us plop in front of the TV or computer in order to "relax" before bed. But electronics are anything but relaxing. The bright lights and sounds stimulate your brain and increase physical stress. And, as most of us know from firsthand experience, TV usually delays sleep—"I must see the ending of the episode!" So do yourself a favor and turn off the electronics at least half an hour before sleep.

5. **Get in Bed:** Spend the last half of the Restorative Hour in bed. Make your bedroom a relaxing, comfortable space; after all, your bed should only have three purposes: reading, sleeping, and doing the horizontal polka (if you know what I mean . . .). Don't pay bills in bed, argue with your partner in bed, or do work in bed. When you keep your bed a stress-free zone, your brain immediately knows it's time to relax when you get under the covers.

Attitude influence isn't just for the morning; practice positive thinking and deep breathing before bed as well. "I will have a restorative and restful sleep" is a helpful mantra for those who suffer from insomnia or nightmares. You could also pray—or simply practice gratitude—during this period.

Healthy Tipping Point Success Story: Tina, 27, Georgia

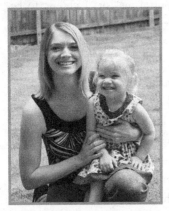

It started while I was in college, living at home to save money. My relationship with my father was emotionally grueling, and as a result, I tried to make myself feel better by controlling my food. Then, one night, I had an "extra" spoonful of peanut butter, which turned into half the jar. Crying hysterically, I grabbed my brother's box of Pop-Tarts and proceeded to eat them all.

That was my first binge. I endured many, many more during the next five years. Whenever I had a hard day, I turned to food. I would stop at the store on the way home from work and buy candies, cookies, baked goods, or ice-cream sandwiches, and I would eat the entire box on my drive home. An entire day's worth of calories—gone in twenty minutes or less.

Of course, bingeing only made me feel more stressed out, which meant the bingeing cycle would often continue for days on end. Afterward, I would restrict food to compensate. I also labeled foods as "good" or "bad," which ended up making me feel deprived because I always focused on what I couldn't have. I was very good at hiding the evidence of my binges and crash diets, and no one, not even my husband, knew what I was going through for so long.

I never told anyone because I saw it as my biggest weakness. I felt so embarrassed that I couldn't overcome the bingeing. Also, on some subconscious level, I didn't want to tell anyone—especially my husband—because I knew that telling him would make me accountable to overcoming the problem. Part of me *wanted* to binge. It was a form of addiction for me, a way to deal with my emotions.

I began to hate myself. I couldn't control my behavior, and I felt myself becoming depressed. I didn't want to go back to that dark place, so I focused on growing my faith. I took time each morning to pray or meditate, repeating over and over, "God, help me love myself like you love me. Help me see I am, in fact, worth something." Whenever I felt stressed, I would focus on positive thoughts like, "Food does not control me" or "I choose to be healthy." Telling my husband about my struggles also helped, too. I'm so glad I found the courage to tell him because he was extremely supportive and understanding.

Then—I became pregnant. I didn't want to harm my developing baby through my bad habits. And after my daughter was born, I wanted to set a good example and change my habits. Once I had the motivation to change and let go of my strict food rules and feelings of denial and shame, I could consistently make healthier choices. I developed positive coping mechanisms for my stress, like talking to my husband about my feelings, making a cup of tea, or writing a blog post. Blogging helped me realize that I was not alone—bingeing is often such a hush-hush topic, yet so many people can relate.

It's important that you believe in your own worth and set aside time each day to care for your health. Making small, healthy decisions consistently adds up over time to a healthy and happier you. If you slip up and experience a bout of emotional eating, just return to normal eating as quickly as possible. Don't try to compensate by restricting; just learn from the experience and move on. Respect yourself by eating well and eating enough. Do not put yourself down—you deserve more.

Two

DEVELOPING A HEALTHY
RELATIONSHIP WITH YOUR
BODY AND FOOD

Once I reach my goal weight, I'll go on that tropical holiday."

"When I firm up, I'll finally feel comfortable enough to shower with my spouse."

"Someday, I'll lose this pregnancy weight, and I'll wear sleeveless shirts again."

"When I can finally run a ten-minute mile, I'll enter that 5K."

Too often, we put our lives—and our self-love—on hold until the "someday" occurs. Maybe we don't feel entirely comfortable enough with our physical appearance. Or maybe we're not ready to expose our deep, dark emotions to the world. Perhaps we fear that we'll be judged by other people. So instead of trying new things and embracing life, we pull back, waiting until we're 100 percent confident we're "ready."

The funny thing about the Myth of the Someday is that our "someday" never seems to really come. Maybe we do reach our goal weight or run faster, but we still feel closed off and scared. Our someday gets pushed back. And back. And it will continue to get pushed back, far in the future, because the real issue isn't what we look like or what other people think about us . . . the trouble lies within. If you struggle with body acceptance or disordered eating, you may also struggle to define long-term goals that are not appearance based, which sets yourself up for failure and stalls out your quest for a true Healthy Tipping Point. That's because problems with accepting your body and with eating issues are the Myth of the Someday's ultimate obstacles, keeping your focus on physical matters and off personal growth.

> Stop buying into the Myth of the Someday. Proactively seek out happiness and acceptance *today*.

This someday type of thinking is so limiting; it literally squeezes your self-esteem to death. There is no legitimate reason to put off your own happiness. You are good enough right now. You are wonderfully and uniquely made. You are worthy of respect and love, and if you don't have those things in your life, you owe it to yourself to go out and find them.

Does this mean we shouldn't seek to improve ourselves? That we should sit on the couch and eat mini cupcakes all day long? Of course not! Self-improvement, learning, developing new skills and abilities, and exploring the range of your physical and mental gifts are part of being a human being. The trouble occurs when you don't believe you're good enough to enjoy your body, your relationships, your life . . . right now. Not someday. Now!

When you put your life off until someday, you take a terrible, terrible risk: someday might never come. Literally—you might not live to rock that bikini on the beach or scrub your husband down in the shower. We are merely mortals, flesh and blood that is so fragile in comparison to our big, beautiful souls. And although it sounds like a platitude, it's completely true—one day, your life will flash before your eyes, and you better make sure the show is worth watching.

The most amazing side effect of a healthy relationship with your mind and body is that it creates an unstoppable force of momentum in your life.

Taking steps to cultivate self-esteem will spill over into all areas of your life, and you'll find it easier to stick with all types of healthy habits.

Life is for living; what are you waiting for?

Rock What You've Got

Our nation is suffering from a severe—and sometimes deadly—body-acceptance crisis. So many of us are so ashamed by our bodies that we withdraw from life activities, like going out with friends, speaking up at work, or even exercising because we're afraid of being judged. Fifty-four percent of women would rather be hit by a truck than be fat. And 81 percent of ten-year-old girls say they are "afraid" of becoming fat.[3] On average, women engage in thirteen negative body thoughts *a day*—nearly one for every waking hour of life. And this issue is certainly not limited to girls and women—approximately 10 percent of anorexics and 40 percent of people struggling with binge eating disorder are male.[4]

HOW BODY CONFIDENT ARE YOU?

Body-acceptance issues can be so sneaky and pervasive that we often don't even realize how toxic our thoughts are—they just seem to be "normal." Read over the following statements—do you see yourself in any of them?

"I weigh myself more often than I would like. I feel compulsive about stepping on the scale."

"I catch myself squeezing parts of my body, like my stomach or thighs, and thinking about how big they are."

"Getting dressed to go out is always a challenge because I feel like nothing looks right on me."

"I find myself comparing my body to others' frequently."

> "I don't want people to think I'm full of myself, so I put myself down. I can't let myself feel good about my appearance."
>
> "The scale holds a lot of control over me. If the number is down, I am happy. If it is up, I feel very upset."
>
> "How I feel about my body wavers constantly. I might think I look pretty good in the morning, but by the end of the day, I feel so unattractive."

Fat Talk is the primary symptom of our body-acceptance crisis. It is negative self-talk about your appearance (or abilities). Fat Talk sounds like this: "My thighs are so huge; I look like a whale," "I'm so embarrassed to wear a bathing suit at the beach," "He'll/she'll never like me because of how I look," or "I am disgusting." These self-put-downs are so incredibly common in our everyday discourse that we tend to gloss over the statements, thinking that it's not a big deal to say, think, or hear such things. But it is a big deal—a really big deal. Fat Talk slowly chips away at our self-esteem and taints our relationships, our professional careers, and even our physical health. And when you Fat Talk in front of others, you project this negativity onto your friends—and they're left wondering, "If she thinks she's so ugly, what does she think about *me*?"

Why are we so hard on ourselves? Why do we treat ourselves so harshly?

THE SOURCE OF THE CRISIS

As it relates to body acceptance, the Myth of the Someday goes a little something like this: "Someday, when I am skinny/have bigger boobs/get rid of this disgusting gut/figure out how to cover up this patch of thinning hair/don't have cellulite, I will be happy." It's all about your appearance. Everything is based on how you—or others—see your body. If you could wave a magic wand and change your appearance, as the myth goes, you'd be happy.

Have you ever checked yourself out in the mirror, thought you looked pretty good, and then headed out, strutting confidently until you hear an insensitive remark or catch an unflattering glimpse of yourself in the mirror? All your confidence comes crashing down. The Myth of the Someday assumes that our body-acceptance issues are solely about our physical appearance. The thought process is inherently flawed. After all, body-acceptance levels can fluctuate so rapidly—sky-high one moment and beat down the next—without a physical change in appearance. That's because there's something deeper going on, something under the skin and in your heart.

Your self-esteem (and therefore, your body acceptance) is highly influenced by your thoughts, relationships, and experiences.

The people in your early life, such as your parents, siblings, first loves, and friends, had an especially profound impact on your baseline esteem levels. If you were raised in an emotionally balanced household and generally treated in a loving, caring way, you probably view yourself in a more positive light than someone who did not feel valued as a child. If you grew up in an unstable household and others' behaviors signaled to you that you were not worth listening to or respecting, you may struggle with low self-worth, even as an adult. Even if childhood was decades ago, the negative experiences of being bullied, abused, or simply ignored as a young child or teen will stay with you if you do not actively work to untangle your emotions about your past.

Our adult relationships also have a profound impact on our self-esteem. If you surround yourself with people who tell you that you're not "worth it" or believe they aren't worth it, either, your self-esteem will suffer. Toxic attitudes roll over you like dark clouds, blocking out the sun and making everything seem dark and gloomy.

Another factor at play is our society's definition of beauty and attractiveness. As briefly touched on earlier, our society has a very limited view of what is considered acceptable, for both women and men. This message is reinforced through magazines, television shows, movies, books, cultural norms, and direct experiences with other people. Put your body-image issues in a larger context—where did you first learn what is an "ideal shape" for a woman and a man? Why do you think teeth have to be perfectly straight to be attractive? Why do you feel compelled to wear makeup or always dress in a certain style? As a child, did you watch a movie or over-hear something that strongly shaped your views on beauty?

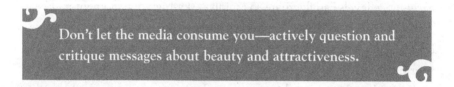

Don't let the media consume you—actively question and critique messages about beauty and attractiveness.

Women have made so much social progress during the last one hundred years. We won the right to vote; we earned the legal right to equal pay. Sexual assault within a marriage is now a crime—yes, for a very long time, it was *actually* legal for a husband to rape a wife. We can work outside of the home without being socially shunned. And yet, there are still pervasive, backward social attitudes about women that plague our society at the deep-est level. More often than not, especially in the media, a woman's worth boils down to whether she is "hot" or not.

When Hillary Rodham Clinton ran for president of the United States in 2008, much attention was paid to the way she dressed and acted—either she was too "butch," dressing like a man in pantsuits, or too feminine, having the gall to cry in public. In January 2007, a *New York Times* piece lambasted Clinton for wearing "a long parade of unflattering outfits and unnervingly changing hairdos" as First Lady.[5] Can you even imagine such an article being written about a male politician? Of course not. Women, even women of incredible intellectual and political power, are trivialized by the media. What matters most, the media implies, is a woman's appearance—her hair, her outfit, her mannerisms. What she says is secondary to whether she looks "right" saying it.

Whether our culture is lampooning a female politician for being unat-tractive or devoting centerfold displays to the best celebrity bikini bodies, the message is loud and clear: appearance matters, above all else. It doesn't matter if you're smart enough to become secretary of state; our society wants to know if you're hiding cellulite under that pantsuit.

In fact, appearance matters so much that the media and marketers take matters into their own hands, wielding tools like Photoshop to make so many celebrities look picture perfect. Now, Photoshop isn't inherently evil—it can be used to lighten or darken images, create neat special effects, and remove unsightly boogers from a bride's nose. But too often, marketers use Photoshop to make models and celebrities appear absolutely flawless, digitally removing love handles, wrinkles, pimples, and cellulite; lengthening necks and legs; pumping up hair thickness; and increasing eye, biceps, and breast size.

Above all else, our society—both in the media and in real life—is obsessed with thinness. So marketers will Photoshop female celebrities and models to conform to the very rigid, extremely unrealistic, and dangerously unhealthy Thin Ideal (one study determined that 70 percent of *Playboy* centerfolds—long considered by many men and women to represent the ideal female form—weighed 15 percent less than their ideal healthy weight!).[6] Marketers will digitally manipulate men to conform to the Muscular Ideal, a physical shape characterized by low body fat and lots of bulging muscles, as well as perfectly straight, white teeth and a head of glossy, thick hair.

The problem, of course, is that these Photoshopped ideals aren't just unhealthy—they are actually unobtainable. The Thin and Muscular Ideals are a caricature of beauty. And yet, because the messaging is so pervasive, these ideals are the ruler by which we measure our own appearance.

Constantly looking at photographs and seeing commercials that depict women and men as the Thin Ideal and Muscular Ideal have damaged our collective body acceptance. Seven out of ten young girls say they want to look like a character on television, and most women (68 percent) say that they feel badly about themselves after reading fashion magazines. Whether consciously or not, women are constantly comparing themselves to the Thin Ideal; as a result, 75 percent of healthy-weight women think they are overweight, and 90 percent of women overestimate their own body size![7]

KIDS' PLAY

Much ado is made about Barbie's unrealistic proportions; if Barbie were real, she'd be six foot nine inches tall and have a forty-inch bust and twenty-inch waist. But a popular boys' toy—GI Joe—creates similarly unhealthy expectations for little boys. If GI Joe was real, he'd be five foot ten inches and have twenty-seven-inch biceps and a fifty-five-inch chest (the 1964 version of the toy would have twelve-inch biceps and a forty-four-inch chest). When Arnold Schwarzenegger was at the peak of his bodybuilding career, his biceps were twenty-two inches and his chest was fifty-seven inches.[8] What messages are we sending our children with toys that promote such unrealistic standards?

Why would the media and marketers promote body ideals that are damaging us physically and emotionally? It's all about the bottom line. Marketers *want* you to feel badly about yourself. That's right—they want you to suffer from low body acceptance. If you lack self-esteem, you'll look to outside sources—like beauty products—to feel better about yourself. Marketers know that we aren't going to shell out twenty-five dollars for antiwrinkle cream unless we are convinced that aging is inherently unattractive. So they use tricks like Photoshop to make us question our worth and try to fill the empty void inside with products.

If you suffer from body-acceptance issues, know that the anxiety is about more than your appearance—your personal history and our society's attitudes are involved, too. As an extension of this mind-body connection, we should also acknowledge that body-acceptance issues don't discriminate; you can suffer from low self-esteem and be big, tall, short, male, female, skinny, blond, brunette, flat-chested, hairy, or muscular. To think, "That girl can't have any real problems—she's so pretty!" minimizes the complexity of body-image issues. After all, there is much more to body acceptance than appearance. You can't look at someone and see their family history, the impact of media expectations, or their mental health struggles. The only thing we wear on the outside is our clothes. Everything else requires a deeper look.

MOVING TOWARD ACCEPTANCE

Whatever you look like, you deserve love and respect, from yourself and from others. You can be working toward a healthy weight loss and still have body acceptance. These two concepts are not inherently contradictory. True self-esteem isn't dependent on what you look like. You can *accept* and *appreciate* your body no matter where you are on your healthy journey.

Your self-worth should not wait for "someday." You deserve to be happy right now.

Take a moment to consider: What do you currently base your self-worth on? Who decides if you're "good enough"? Your family? Your partner? The media? Acknowledging that these definitions of worth may be tainted or toxic is the first step to moving toward body acceptance. These outside sources try to define your worth, but the reality is that the only definition of your worth that actually matters is your own. Free yourself from focusing solely on the outside—you'll never get anywhere significant by focusing on appearance.

HEALTHY BODY ACCEPTANCE

If you've been struggling to change the way you look and are suffering from low self-esteem as a result, maybe it's time to simply focus on changing the way you treat yourself. Healthy body acceptance isn't about believing you're the hottest person in the room; it's about love, appreciation, and forgiveness. Provided below are some healthy body statements. Try using these statements when you encounter negative body-image thoughts.

"I'm not perfect, but that's okay. I'm human."

"My worth is about much more than my body. I'm an amazing friend and a hard worker."

"I am grateful to have a healthy, functioning body that allows me to enjoy my life."

"These lumps, bumps, scars, and wrinkles show how much I've been through—and I'm stronger and stronger every day. I can overcome anything."

"Instead of focusing on what I don't like, I choose to focus on the things I do like and appreciate."

"I will not let our messed-up society's view of beauty influence how I feel about my amazing body."

It is time to change how you react to our society's conversation about ideal body shapes. The conversation includes external voices—like the media, your friends, and your family history—and internal voices—like Fat Talk. Poor body image can be the result of a very one-sided conversation; the external and internal voices are telling you how to feel and treat yourself, but your heart and head aren't talking back. Instead, you're letting others make up the rules and decide your self-worth, even if the standards for your worth are impossible to obtain or unhealthy.

Becoming mentally and physically healthy is all about small changes. Don't feel pressured to overhaul your body acceptance overnight; after all, it took a lifetime for you to develop your self-esteem, and it's unrealistic to expect to change your thought patterns in a few days! Instead, focus on making small, positive steps toward the healthy attitude you'd like to have.

- **Blast Through Limiting Beliefs:** Everyone perceives life through a unique filter of their own experiences. This filter can be positive or negative, depending on your experiences and the specific situation. Perhaps you've never been betrayed by a friend, so your friendship filter is to always trust others. This filter is a positive one that enriches your life and encourages you to develop close relationships with the people around you. Alternatively, you may have experienced several bad breakups and struggle to trust your current partner because you "expect" them to cheat on you. This negative filter damages your happiness and puts a strain on your relationship.

A negative filter creates limiting beliefs, which are destructive thought patterns. A limiting belief holds you back by preventing personal growth and the development of solid, healthy relationships. Examples of body-acceptance limiting beliefs include "I will always be unattractive," "I will never be satisfied with my appearance," "No one will love me until I lose weight," or "Everyone is judging me based on how I look." You become what you think. Buying into toxic thought patterns will influence your behavior, exacerbate low self-esteem, and—ultimately—reinforce your limiting beliefs. If you believe you don't deserve to love your body, perhaps you will continue to punish your body with unhealthy foods . . . and then, you'll feel even worse about yourself and your body.

Slowly create healthier thought patterns by identifying and challenging your negative filter and limiting beliefs. One way to challenge your limiting beliefs is to look for real-world examples that disprove the belief. For example, if you believe no one will love you because of your appearance, remind yourself of couples who love each other unconditionally. Also, note that your limiting beliefs are essentially ultimatums—very black and white. Work to develop beliefs that are more flexible and forgiving. Instead of, "Everyone is judging me based

Lay the foundation for the life you want through your thoughts.

on how I look," consider this new belief: "First impressions matter, but it's about more than my appearance—I'm a friendly and outgoing person, and people will like me because of this."

- **Crush the Fat Talk:** As you alter limiting beliefs, you will naturally cut down on external and internal Fat Talk. Stopping negative self-talk is extremely important, since Fat Talk has a strong impact on your self-esteem. Like limiting beliefs, Fat Talk is a self-fulfilling prophecy; if you talk down to yourself, you will struggle to make healthier choices because you'll believe you don't deserve to.

  To halt Fat Talk, first acknowledge that you are engaging in the behavior. Fat Talkers engage in the habit for many reasons: it's socially acceptable and expected (women often Fat Talk as a bonding mechanism, for example); it's habitual; and it's a coping mechanism for stress and low self-esteem. Fat Talk is so common that many Fat Talkers don't even realize they are doing it. Pay attention to your thoughts and words, and when you catch yourself Fat Talking, consciously correct the toxic activity. If you Fat Talked in your head, identify the behavior and redirect your thoughts to something more positive. If you Fat Talked aloud, correct yourself in the conversation; your Fat Talk can have a negative impact on whoever hears it. You can say, "I shouldn't talk down to myself like that."

  Replace the Fat Talk with a positive but realistic thought. But you must believe the new thought! For example, if you just Fat Talked about the size of your thighs, it might not be helpful to think, "I am a freakin' supermodel!" A more effective positive thought may be, "I don't like the way these shorts fit, but my legs are amazing because they carried me across a 5K finish line!"

  The most common Fat Talk phrase is, "I feel so fat." But fat isn't an emotion. There is always something deeper behind Fat Talk; it's not really about your appearance at all. It's about how you feel about yourself and your situation. If you catch yourself Fat Talking, ask what's really going on. When you question yourself, you may be surprised to discover that you don't feel "fat"—you feel nervous, ashamed, guilty, unhappy, or mad. Honor your true emotions!

OPERATION BEAUTIFUL

Can one Post-it note change the way you see yourself? OperationBeautiful .com believes so! Operation Beautiful promotes posting positive messages— such as "You are beautiful, inside and out" or "Take a diet from negative thoughts, fill yourself with positive ones!"—in random public places, like public bathroom mirrors, on the gym scale, and in library books. Posting the notes reinforces positive thinking and encourages a focus on the healthy ideal. For more information, check out my new book *Operation Beautiful: Transforming the Way You See Yourself One Post-It Note at a Time* or my Web site, www.OperationBeautiful.com. If you want to share the message with a young girl in your life, send her a copy of *Operation Beautiful for Best Friends*.

- **Become a Critical Consumer:** Take a good, hard look at your media consumption—do you read any magazines or watch any television shows that always leave you feeling miserable and low? Why torture yourself? Choose to engage in media that uplifts and inspires you— not media that makes you feel terrible about yourself and your body. Cancel that subscription or change the channel.

  When you encounter an image or article that stirs up negative thoughts, take a moment to consider why you feel this way. Is the piece trying to make you feel bad to motivate you to buy something? Is the advertisement reinforcing gender or social stereotypes? Is the model Photoshopped to conform to the Thin Ideal or Muscular Ideal? Sure signs of Photoshopping include lack of wrinkles or pores; golden, glowing skin; necks or legs that seem impossibly long; no "jutting out" along the hip line; extremely cut muscles; and body parts that don't line up. (For example, a model is sitting behind a table, but her upper body and lower body are at an impossible angle, indicating her waist has been "shaved down.")

- **Focus on Health, Not Size:** As it relates to body acceptance, your limiting beliefs and Fat Talk, as well as the messaging in the media, boil down to one thing: a focus on the Thin Ideal (or the Muscular Ideal). Remember, the Thin Ideal isn't just about being skinny; it's about being physically perfect in every single way.

  Work to change your thought patterns to focus on being healthy, not perfect. The Healthy Ideal looks different on different people; after all, healthy bodies come in a variety of shapes and sizes. This balanced ideal is about enjoying delicious, wholesome foods and yummy treats; working out because it makes you feel good; and prioritizing mental health. The Healthy Ideal is about forgiveness and acceptance. It's about celebrating life—not restricting it. The Healthy Ideal doesn't require perfection. The Healthy Ideal focuses only on positive progress.

  If you're making small efforts to become the happiest, mentally and physically healthiest person possible, you're discovering your Healthy Ideal and are well on your way to your Healthy Tipping Point. The Healthy Ideal is a fluid and forgiving way to look at your body and your health. If you embrace the message of the Healthy Ideal, you can accept your body right now. You don't have to wait until "someday." You can love yourself in this very moment. Give yourself a mental hug—you're worth it.

> Ditch the Thin Ideal or the Muscular Ideal and focus on the Healthy Ideal, which looks different for different people.

Freeing Yourself from Disordered Eating

Food is fuel—but it's also so much more. It's birthday cake, Thanksgiving turkey, daily coffee rituals, popcorn at the movies. Food is memories and love. Most of our society's social events revolve around eating. Food is, in so many ways, life.

Food and life are so tightly intertwined, it's not surprising that many of our food issues have nothing to do with fiber intake or artificial sweeteners. The tricky part of food is often how we feel about it. Generally speaking, Americans have an extremely negative attitude toward food and its impact on our appearance. As a result, we derive much less pleasure from eating than, say, the French. In one study, Americans were asked what comes to mind upon hearing certain words. Americans were most likely to associate "chocolate cake" with "guilt," and "heavy cream" with "unhealthy." The French said "celebration" when thinking of chocolate cake and "whipped" when imaging heavy cream. Our negative attitude toward food is . . . well, it's pretty depressing (especially considering that the world is full of people starving to death).

Food issues comprise a wide, varied spectrum. At one end are clinically defined eating disorders, such as bulimia (binging and purging through vomiting, laxatives, or extreme exercise); anorexia (restriction of food in order to maintain a low weight, and an all-consuming fear of gaining weight); and binge-eating disorder (characterized by frequent episodes of eating large amounts of food in a short period of time without a compensatory behavior, like purging, accompanied by feelings of shame and guilt). There is also an unspecified eating disorder, where you may not meet the diagnosis criteria for the other, defined disorders.

If you suspect that you may meet the criteria for these disorders, please seek out professional help. A registered dietitian, psychologist, or medical doctor specializing in eating disorders will be able to help. Find experts in your area through an Internet search or ask for a referral from someone you trust. If the first professional you ask for help doesn't give you what you need, try someone else. You deserve a proper evaluation, diagnosis, and treatment plan. Keep asking until you find someone who can help you sort through your disorder. Eating disorders are very serious, potentially life threatening, and can quickly spiral out of control. Even if you think you have things "under control," you should make sure a qualified expert performs an evaluation. It is common for people with eating disorders to think they are in control of their behaviors when they really aren't.

At the other end of the food-issues spectrum is distorted eating. Many people struggle with a negative attitude toward food, but they don't think anything is "wrong" because they do not fit the criteria for a clinical food disorder. And many distorted eating habits—like Fat Talking—are so common that we don't even recognize them as negative behaviors.

Symptoms of distorted eating include (but are certainly not limited to):

- Restriction of food, including delaying eating even though you're hungry;
- Fear/avoidance of certain "unhealthy" or "bad" foods or food groups, like carbohydrates;
- Uncontrollable episodes of eating past the point of fullness;
- Negative self-talk about weight and appearance;
- Compulsively stepping on the scale (most experts recommend, at an absolute maximum, weighing oneself weekly in the morning at the same time of day, and many people choose to only weigh themselves once a month, once a year, or never at all);
- Characterization of foods as either "good" or "bad";
- Use of excessive exercise to "punish" oneself for overeating;
- Feelings of guilt or of not being in control while eating;
- Dislike of eating in public places or in front of other people;
- Guilt or negative emotions after eating "restricted" foods;
- Hyper-focus on planning meals and counting calories;
- Chronic dieting and cycles of weight gain/loss;

- General feelings of being overly sad, anxious, or stressed about food and weight; and
- Frequently thinking about food.

If you identify with any of these symptoms, it's important to know that you do not have to live like this, and you *can* free yourself from these toxic behaviors and actions. Resolving food issues can seem very overwhelming; not only must you alter negative thought patterns, but you must also eliminate negative actions associated with eating. These changes, however, do not need to occur overnight, and progress does not have to be linear. It is natural for your habits to ebb and flow as you move toward balanced living.

And remember—you don't have to be perfect. In fact, you shouldn't even *try* to become a perfect eater! The stress associated with striving for perfection is too great, and your goal will never, ever be accomplished. Perfection is impossible. Instead, work with an expert who can help you discover what healthy and balanced mean for you, in your personal, professional, and spiritual life, as well as how you relate to food. After all, life is food and food is life; there's no untangling the two. To live a happy, full life, you must resolve your issues with food.

- **Stop Restricting:** The first step to overcoming your distorted habits is to stop restricting. Restriction comes in many forms: you may be afraid to eat certain foods; always skip breakfast; or skip dinner if you ate a "big" lunch or didn't exercise. If you deny yourself foods, your body and mind will eventually rebel. Restriction throws your body into a tailspin, a literal biological freak-out, and will trigger an intense binge. Feelings of guilt, sadness, and a lack of control will inevitably follow. After the binge, you'll feel compelled to restrict, which will renew the vicious cycle.

  Restriction has serious emotional and physical consequences, and it certainly does nothing for your overall health. People who restrict their food are more likely to have an episode of overeating, followed by guilt and a desire to "make up" for their "bad" behavior. A healthy body is fueled throughout the day in moderate amounts at regular intervals. Focus on eating three square meals and one or two snacks throughout the day, roughly every three to five hours, which is a typical hunger cycle. If you feel the urge to restrict, ask yourself, "What's really going on here?" Like body acceptance, many distorted eating behaviors are really about something much, much deeper. You may notice that you feel tempted to restrict after a stressful day at work or comparing yourself to someone else, for example.

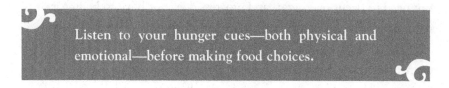

Listen to your hunger cues—both physical and emotional—before making food choices.

- **Eat Intuitively and Honor Your Hunger:** Many of us can't even recognize or distinguish between hunger cues after years and years of yo-yo dieting. We eat when we're "supposed to" and feel guilty if we're hungry in between meals. We've been trained to ignore what our bodies and hearts tell us—and, obviously, we're not mentally or physically healthier as a result! There's a better way to eat: intuitively. What does this mean, exactly? Intuitive eating focuses on allowing your internal hunger cues to "weigh in" before making food choices.

  There are actually two types of hunger cues: physical and emotional cues. Physical hunger cues occur three to five hours after your last meal (although they can occur sooner) and usually are characterized by an empty, grumbling stomach. When you feel physically hungry, you should always eat. If you're between meals, have a snack (see pages 236–38 for a list of healthy snack ideas). And just as you should honor your hunger, try to honor your feelings of fullness, too. Eat your meals slower than you would normally, giving pause toward the end of the meal to check in on your fullness levels.

  Emotional hunger is more complicated. You may feel it when

you're stressed, angry, happy, tired, bored, or anxious. Emotional hunger is accompanied with a sense of compulsion and usually a craving for a particular food. If you think, "I want to eat something," check in to see if you're physically hungry, and if you discover you're actually still quite full from lunch, ask yourself, "Why do I want to eat right now?" Your mind might respond, "I'm bored." This is an example of how your mind uses food as a distraction, an attempt to smother or ignore negative emotions. Emotional overeating (eating to very full) can lead to unhealthy rapid weight gain and other health complications.

But sometimes, emotional eating is okay, and there are many reasons to eat beyond physical hunger—holidays, celebrations, stress, and the simple fact that food is delicious. If you've had a bad day at work, and the thing that will make you relax is a big glass of wine and a slice of chocolate cake, go for it. Before you eat, make a conscious decision to savor and enjoy. Remind yourself not to feel guilty afterward; after all, you made a thoughtful and purposeful decision.

- **Declare a Truce:** If you find yourself labeling foods as "good" or "bad," it's time to declare a truce on food. All foods can be part of a healthy diet, if eaten in moderation and in balance with other nutritious foods. When you hear yourself thinking, "This is bad food," that's the distortion talking.
- **Focus on the Healthy Ideal:** Just as focusing on the Healthy Ideal, not the Thin Ideal, can help you achieve body acceptance, ditching appearance-based thinking can help you overcome distorted eating habits. Diet books and magazines have convinced many of us that we need to eat less than 1,200 calories a day, that we must avoid carbs, that we shouldn't eat dessert—all of this is nonsense! This is restrictive and distorted, thinly veiled as "normal" behaviors.

It's understandable if you feel a bit overwhelmed by the lifestyle changes you want to make to achieve your Healthy Tipping Point, especially if you are grappling with a distorted food outlook. If you focus 90 percent of your diet on real food in reasonable portions, you're doing a great service for your body and mind by finding a sense of balance in your eating habits. Take the time to focus on how delicious real food tastes, and how good it makes you feel, both physically and mentally, to make healthier choices. Make the effort to derive pleasure—not guilt—from eating by doing simple things, like taking the time to set the table properly, eating from pretty dishes, consciously choosing treats instead of mindlessly reaching for them, and identifying what healthy meals and snacks give you an energy boost.

- **Seek Help:** If you suffer from an eating disorder or feelings of distorted eating, please know that you are worth seeking professional help. Repeat: you are worth it! Too many people put off getting assistance for far too long. For more information, check out the National Eating Disorders Association at www.edap.org.

Healthy Tipping Point Success Story: June, 48, Texas

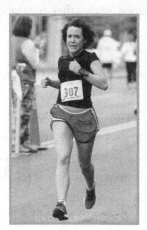

I dabbled in drugs during high school and college. But when I moved to Las Vegas in 1985, it all spiraled out of control. I started using crystal meth. I was a functioning user, which meant I could hold down a steady job and maintain a good reputation while using. I was using about four times a week (Thursday through Sunday) solidly, and this went on for seven years.

My addiction got worse and worse and began to impact my life—I would miss work and skip out on family functions. I was so thin.

I left a man I loved, lost my job, sold my house, and blew through $30,000 from the sale in no time. Then, my father, who I was very close to, passed away after a long fight with cancer.

When I became convinced that I'd kill myself if I kept using, I got clean. I was struggling with some health problems, like unexpected weight gain (which I later found out was due to hypothyroidism), and I needed a healthy outlet for stress, so I decided to start running. In 2005, clean and sober, I ran my first race. I thought it was a 5K run, but when I got there I realized it was actually five *miles*. I finished by run/walking . . . and I never looked back! I did my first half-marathon in October 2006, my first marathon in January 2007, and I'm planning to do my sixth marathon soon.

Bikram and power vinyasa yoga give me a sense of peace that I had never known before. I felt so much more in tune physically, emotionally, and spiritually. I love the way yoga makes me feel. Being in a room surrounded by mirrors forces you to see in a new, more positive light. Yoga truly made me love my body for the vessel that it is!

Here is a story that I've only ever told one other person: this past May, I went to run a 12K race—Bay to Breakers in San Francisco. That night, my girlfriends and I went out and met some guys. One of them pulled me aside and handed me a vial of cocaine to do "for fun." I am going to tell you right now, I almost did it. But I didn't. I gave it back, said good night to my friends, caught a cab, and went to the hotel to prepare for the race. I was so, so proud of myself.

I've gone through a lot—and, in the process, I've rediscovered how strong, healthy, and independent I am. I'm redefining myself. When it comes to eating better or running a marathon, it all comes down to how badly you want to change your life.

Three

FLEXING YOUR
MIND MUSCLE

Every day, we make hundreds of choices. Some choices are small and without consequence. Should I wear a blue shirt or this black shirt? Should I have cream in my coffee? Should I cook dinner or get takeout? But every now and then, we make a choice that creates a divergence in our life path and irrevocably pushes us in another direction. This choice might be small—a matter of being in the right place at the right time (or the wrong place at the wrong time)—or very big. Will I break up with my partner? What job will I take? What city will I live in? It's the big decisions that, in retrospect, have the most visible impact on our life path. We can clearly point to a specific day and say, "Because this happened to me, I am here."

While big decisions seem to have the most powerful impact on your life path, there is an even greater force behind these decisions—your attitude. Day in and day out, your attitude subtly influences your *options*. Just like a magnet with a positive and negative pole, a positive attitude will attract better options, and a negative attitude will push options away.

Your life is probably very crowded right now—work, school, family, friends, and other responsibilities and stressors. And if you want to change, it can be difficult to see where you'll have time for the effort. It is absolutely essential that you adopt a positive, forgiving, and open attitude while searching for your Healthy Tipping Point; this approach will help create the space for success in your life. A positive attitude will attract better options and enable you to make healthier choices. With a negative attitude, your options seem very small and limited.

Proactive and Positive

When you're watching a movie, the sound track usually clues you in to what's going to happen next. Happy, upbeat music tells us the couple is about to kiss or the hero is going to save the day. Brooding, deep tones signal that all hell is about to break loose. Your attitude is the sound track to your life, except the music isn't following a script—it's creating the script as it goes.

Many of us let this sound track play on in the background. We don't try to consciously influence the playlist; we passively listen. As we get dressed, our attitude sings, "Youlookterrible, terrible! *Terrible*! Whyareyou wearing that, wearing that? Whodoyouthinkyouarrrre, who do you think you are!" When we sit down for that pivotal job interview, our attitude wails, "You're gonna fail, fail, FAILLLLLL!" And your attitude foreshadows the outcome—you feel unconfident, unappealing, and stupid. You act unconfident, unappealing, and stupid. The interviewer perceives you as unconfident, unappealing, and stupid.

When you feel negativity brewing, take a deep breath and choose to respond in a proactive, positive, and purposeful way.

Let's not sugarcoat it—it's not easy to change your thought patterns, especially ones that have been ingrained since childhood. Developing a positive attitude is a learning process that evolves and grows over many, many years. Furthermore, a positive attitude is constantly challenged by negative events, and the thinker's ability to remain positive may naturally ebb and flow in response to such stressors.

To change your attitude, you must pay attention to the sound track in your head and consciously make changes to the music. Instead of letting your attitude control you, you must control your attitude. While we cannot control everything that happens to us, and we certainly cannot control other people, controlling your attitude will create more positive options, thereby enabling you to make better, healthier choices. Changing our attitude rewrites the sound track; the scenes of your life end differently.

How do we combat negativity? **Choose to respond in a positive, proactive, and purposeful manner.** Let's break this down because each component of this directive is very important. "Choose to respond" implies that you have the power to control your reaction. Often, we remark that we "got swept up in the moment" or "acted without thinking," but the reality is that you—and you alone—control your reaction to stressful situations.

When we choose to respond in a "proactive, positive, and purposeful manner," we make a conscious effort to alter the melody of our attitude. Imagine that your mind is in Positive Boot Camp. You must instruct your mind to be more positive. When you catch yourself thinking, "I cannot . . ." firmly resolve, "But I can . . ." When you hear your attitude singing, "You are going to fail," croon back, "I am going to try my hardest." Do this in a purposeful manner—truly consider where your negative reaction came from and how a positive attitude will help the situation. And above all else, be proactive with your positive thinking. When you encounter situations that you anticipate will be difficult, begin to pump yourself up in advance. Tell yourself you *can* do it and that the outcome will be successful.

> Life isn't what happens *to* you. Life is what you *do* with the hand you're dealt.

Let's use an example to illustrate why a positive attitude is so important and how you can use it to forge the life you want. You want to develop a healthy exercise routine. You have a detailed short- and long-term plan for success and a stellar source of motivation; however, if you aren't positive, proactive, and purposeful in the face of a challenge, you will soon fall off the wagon. Challenges, after all, are inevitable! You exercise regularly for weeks on end, but your boss is a monster, and your workload flares up. Suddenly, you feel like you have no free time or energy to work out as often as you'd like. If you are not in control of your attitude, this situation will naturally trigger feelings of guilt or anger. This negative attitude would say that it's all or nothing; if you are working out, you are a success, but if you aren't, you are an utter failure. As a result of these negative emotions, your healthy eating habits begin to slide, which triggers another negative reaction, damages your confidence, makes you feel tired and irritable, contributes to your lack of energy, and ensures that, even on a free Saturday afternoon, you'll skip the gym. "What's the point?" sneers your negative attitude.

Do you see what happened here? Your thoughts became a runaway train, gaining speed until you careened off the tracks. All it took was one trying circumstance—a busier work schedule—and everything fell to pieces . . . because you believed it would.

To cultivate a healthier attitude, you must choose to respond proactively, positively, and purposefully. You could think, "Work sure is getting busy. Instead of committing to five workouts a week, I'll commit to two until my workload lightens up. If I do three or four, I'll be really proud of myself." By anticipating challenges and managing your own expectations, you are being proactive. You could also remind yourself, "Any workout is a good workout. My body is already taxed from spending so much time at work; it's better not to push myself at the gym. I should work out only when I have the energy." This is putting a positive spin on the situation. Last, you could think, "I'm so stressed right now. What I don't need is a bad attitude. Instead, I'm going to recommit to taking time for myself during the Power Hour. I'm also going to plan active social events so I can exercise while seeing my friends on the weekend." By identifying solutions and adjusting your goals, you are being purposeful in your reaction to the situation.

All thoughts, actions, and events are connected to one another; choosing to be proactive, positive, and purposeful in your thoughts will create a happier, more positive life. All events in your life can be spun in a positive or negative light; each experience is a learning opportunity.

A New Spin on Self-Doubt

If you find yourself believing that you can't do it, don't deserve it, or just aren't good enough, you're experiencing a moment of self-doubt. Our self-doubt can come from body-acceptance issues, distorted eating habits, fear of judgment by others, or worry over finances and success. It's okay to have moments of self-doubt—it makes you human! Occasionally questioning and comparing yourself to others is normal.

Self-doubt has the potential to be tremendously powerful. And like most things in life, this power can be harnessed and used for good or evil. Self-doubt can consume and paralyze you, prevent you from making healthy choices, or contribute to a negative attitude.

Flip self-doubt around and use it as a powerful motivator.

On the other hand, self-doubt can be the fuel to your fire. It's helpful to think of whisperings of doubt inside your mind as a *challenge*. When your mind says, "You can't do that," scream back, "Yes I can! Wanna make a bet?" Show the self-doubt who is the boss—YOU! If you try something that self-doubt said you were too weak to attempt, you've won. If you fail at something self-doubt predicted you'd bomb, but you try again, you beat self-doubt.

Another way to beat self-doubt is to recognize that life—especially healthy living—is not black and white. There is no "right way" to do everything. The voice of self-doubt is very similar to that of perfectionism. "If you're not going to be perfect, why try at all?" these voices whisper. This, of course, is a ludicrous sentiment. Three steps forward and two steps back is still one step in the direction of your dreams.

Self-doubt wants you to surrender when the going gets tough, but a healthy attitude rebuffs this illogical, black-and-white thinking by reframing goals. The next time you feel doubtful of your abilities, consider your goals and adjust them as necessary to ensure *some* type of success. You never want to set yourself up to fail. Lowering expectations does not mean you will achieve less; you may find that lower expectations take the pressure off, alleviate self-doubt, and allow you to grow and thrive past the point of your original goal. Furthermore, whisperings of self-doubt often have a kernel of truth in them and, if you pay attention, can actually help you create more achievable and beneficial goals.

For example, if you're training for a half-marathon and the training plan is too difficult to keep up with, self-doubt might tell you that you're *never* going to finish the race. You could readjust your goals by switching training plans to something that is a better match for your body. Also, you could acknowledge that you've been struggling with the long runs and decide that, instead of running the entire time, you'll use the walk/run method during the race.

Challenging Your Stress Response

Stress is an unavoidable fact of life. Any time we take on more responsibility or encounter a problem, our stress levels skyrocket. But stress can come from exciting or happy events, too. Getting a promotion, hosting a party, or falling in love are positive examples of stress.

Your body cannot distinguish between good stress and bad stress—it just perceives a stressful situation. Even if the source of the stress is positive or the outcome of the event is positive, stress imparts a tremendous impact. Your body releases a cocktail of powerful hormones, including adrenaline and cortisol, in response to the stressor. These hormones turn on the body and prime it for quick action. Your heart pounds, blood pressure increases, and muscles tighten; your senses become sharper and more focused. These chemicals can be useful in many ways, motivating you to work harder, move faster, and think more creatively. But the stress response, if strong and constant, slowly taxes your mind and body, causing anxiety, headaches, weight gain or loss, back pain, depression, and a weakened immune system.

It's not always possible to eliminate major stress from your life. You can't just storm into your boss's office and yell, "I hate you! You cause stress! I'm quitting!" Well, you *could*, but such an impromptu resignation might only increase stress in the long run.

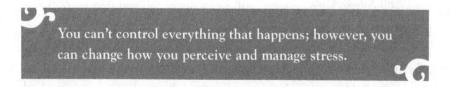

You can't control everything that happens; however, you can change how you perceive and manage stress.

Too often we try to bury stress, piling "other stuff" on top of it to ignore the bad feelings. Negative coping mechanisms are behavioral patterns used to deal with and process stress; examples include working overtime, eating too much or too little, abusing alcohol (my old negative coping mechanism of choice), gambling, smoking cigarettes, shopping, overexercising, sinking into denial or depression, or sleeping excessively. These coping mechanisms often feel really *good* in the moment, which is why we turn to them. A box of cookies tastes pretty wonderful after a terrible day at work. But negative coping mechanisms create additional problems and increase general stress. After all, if you wake up with a raging sugar hangover, you won't feel ready to tackle another workday, and your stress levels will rise again.

You can only change how you perceive and manage stress. Positive coping mechanisms put the power back in your hands, helping you deal with stress in a productive and healthy way. The tricky thing about positive coping mechanisms is most of us don't naturally turn to these methods. Just as we must make an effort to tackle life in a positive, proactive, and purposeful way, we must also make small choices each day to utilize positive coping mechanisms when confronted with stress.

The most effective way to tackle stress is through mental and physical positive coping mechanisms, which are described below:

- **Breathe It Out:** In stressful situations, most people revert to upper chest breathing, which is very shallow and provides the brain with less oxygen. Make an effort to breathe deeply, from your abdomen, when feelings of tension arise. To aid in deep breathing, lie on your back if possible (otherwise, sit tall in a chair) and place your hand below your belly button, feeling your stomach rise and fall as you breathe deeply and in a controlled manner. Silently count to five for each inhale and exhale. Imagine the stress melting away from your body with each exhale.

- **Progressive Relaxation:** Stress typically manifests in your muscles, creating painful little knots. To release your body and relax your mind, lie on your back and tense every single muscle in your body, from your toes to your nose. Clench your fist, flex your calves, and tighten your rear. Hold this total body contraction for ten seconds, and then begin to slowly relax each muscle, one at a time, beginning with your feet. Feel your feet release, then your legs, butt, back, stomach, arms, and neck and face. Combine with deep breathing and repeat several times, if necessary.

- **Meditation:** Meditation has a bad reputation. But it doesn't have to be strenuous, time-consuming, or boring; meditation can be whatever you want it to be! Begin by taking five minutes during the Power Hour or Restorative Hour to simply breathe deeply and quiet your mind. If you struggle to silence your thoughts because your stress level is so high, try visualization. This will give you something relaxing to focus on. For the Happy Place visualization, imagine a relaxing place (a lake house, a beach, a quiet field of wildflowers) and "feel" the location with as many senses as possible. What does the beach smell like? How does the wind feel on your skin? What can you hear? For the Smoke visualization, imagine a cleansing white smoke seeping into your lungs with each deep breath. Imagine the smoke pushing through your entire body, filling you from head to toe, denser and denser with each inhale. Once the smoke surrounds every part of your body, begin to disperse it with each exhale. Imagine that all your negative emotions cling to the smoke and are transported out of your body. If your attention starts to wander during a meditation or visualization, gently bring your thoughts back to the task at hand.

- **See Success:** In anticipation of a stressful event, like a race or a presentation at work, take a moment to visualize success. Run through each step of the entire event in your mind, imagining that everything goes smoothly. If you have to confront a difficult person, imagine the situation in a humorous way. Put your boss in a clown suit or your ex in footie pajamas.

- **Does It Really Matter?:** In the midst of a stressful situation, ask yourself, "Will this matter in a week? Six months? A year?" Many of our stressors aren't *that* big of a deal—a traffic jam, a tiff with a friend. Acknowledging that the stressor really doesn't matter in the grand scheme of life can be so powerful because it thwarts the power of the stress. If the stress is significant, identifying it as such allows you to separate the "real" stress from the "everyday" stress. This process also validates your feelings and focuses your attention on what really matters.

- **Exercise:** Exercise is an excellent way to release feelings of anger or frustration. When negative feelings arise, head out for a long walk or a light jog. Be sure not to work out to the point of exhaustion; this will only put further stress on your body. Healthy exercise should invigorate, not exhaust you.

- **Clean Up:** If your mind is cluttered, organizing your house or desk can help chase away those negative emotions. Do a fifteen-minute pickup. Set a timer and clean as much as you can, taking care to tidy up surface areas that are readily visible (like your dining room table).

- **Draw Boundaries:** Unnecessary stress occurs when you say "yes"— even when you don't have the time or energy to help out. Saying "no" can be very difficult, especially if you identify yourself as a helper or go-to friend. But you'll be no real help to anyone if you're emotionally tapped out. If someone wants you to do something that will increase your stress, buy time by saying, "Let me think about it and get back to you." Step back and consider how saying "yes" will impact your general well-being. It's healthy—and necessary—to put yourself first sometimes or delegate responsibility.

  Drawing boundaries doesn't just relate to your time; toxic people in our life try to monopolize our emotions and energy. You cannot control other people, but you can control how you react to energy vampires. If you don't believe you deserve respect right now—regardless of your past, appearance, or abilities—odds are high that you will engage in self-sabotage or negative coping mechanisms. Demand that other people treat you kindly. And if they don't, stepping back might be the healthiest thing you ever do.

Activities such as baking, traveling, playing with a pet, writing, reading a book, going out to eat, learning a new skill, going to church, stretching or yoga, gardening, or volunteering are other examples of positive coping mechanisms.

Four

TYING IT ALL TOGETHER

Healthy living is about more than diet and exercise. What goes on in your mind and heart is far more important than what you put on your plate or whether you hit the gym. If you're seeking your Healthy Tipping Point moment, a healthy, balanced attitude is a powerful catalyst that accelerates positive changes, making them more powerful and permanent.

Just as you shouldn't expect your body to transform overnight, don't pressure yourself to be emotionally "perfect" all the time. It's not easy to create new thought patterns and behavioral responses, but everything you go through has a grander purpose. There is meaning in all that we experience, if you just look hard enough. Somewhere, underneath all the pressure, stress, and emotional baggage, is the truth: you are amazing. You are incredible. You can do anything you want.

Sometimes, it's just a matter of getting out of your own way.

Healthy Tipping Point Success Story: Rachel, 24, New York

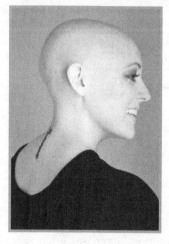

One day, I found a hard, painless lump the size of an olive on my collarbone. Part of me knew it was cancer. However, another small part of me thought, "No way, I'm only twenty-three."

Because I didn't have health insurance through my job yet, I went to a cheap clinic for tests. I was so naïve at the time and didn't know how to fight for the type of medical care that I needed. I had no other symptoms besides the lump, and the doctors brushed it off like it was nothing.

But within a few weeks, I soon started to feel even worse. I had a stabbing pain in my left lung, walking up the subway stairs left me fatigued, my appetite disappeared. I developed so many lumps in my neck and collarbone area that the right side looked like I had a bunch of grapes underneath my skin.

I finally got proper medical insurance and went to see an oncologist. I was sitting in the office, all alone, when I learned that it was most likely lymphoma. The oncologist suggested that I go to the ER and complain of chest pains so I could cut through my insurance's red tape, which would require a two-week wait before a biopsy, and get the immediate help he knew I needed. At the ER, the doctors discovered my heart and lungs were filled with fluid, and I was eventually diagnosed with stage IV non-Hodgkin's lymphoma. I went in for my biopsy and didn't leave for three weeks.

It was frustrating to know that I was initially misdiagnosed, and the cancer built up in my chest for many months. It's so important to be your own advocate when something is wrong with your health and to seek out doctors who will listen and help you. I'm not sure what would have happened if I had gone another two weeks with that fluid around my heart and lungs. My oncologist saved my life because he was so proactive in getting me treated immediately.

Before I was diagnosed, I felt like I had to do it all—work two jobs, maintain a social life, go to the gym, and more. It was exhausting. Being a cancer patient really made me take a look at my life and realize that living isn't all about working and saving money, it's not about going to the gym to burn calories, and it's definitely not about doing things that make you unhappy. As difficult as cancer is, I wouldn't skip any of the challenges I've gone through. I have so much more clarity about what truly matters in life and what doesn't. Often, young people take their health for granted and feel so invincible. I don't anymore.

Cancer taught me many things about life, but I didn't let it rule my life. I just finished my last chemotherapy treatment, and I can safely say that thanks to the disease, I have fallen back in love with my life.

Part II

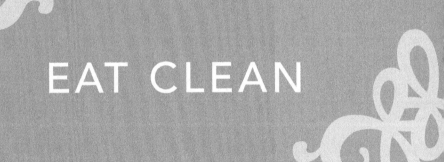

EAT CLEAN

Five

FOOD AS FUEL

E ating can easily become a mindless action. Open mouth, shovel in food, and move on with the day, tackling the dozens of other tasks you need to accomplish. Food can be a source of pleasure, a centerpiece of family events and social outings, or a hobby. It can also be an addiction, a disorder, a crutch, or a weapon. Many of us focus only on the pleasurable effects of eating—"This chocolate cake is so delicious, I'm going to have another slice!"—or the negative emotions we've conditioned ourselves to associate with food—"I feel so guilty after eating that cake!"

We began to unravel the complex relationship between our emotions and food in the "Get Real" section. While part of *your* healthy journey may be to untangle from your emotional issues with food, *everyone* needs to find a way to balance their healthy eating goals with the rest of their life. To make healthy eating really work—at your dinner table, at your job, with kids, at school—you need to strike a balance between caring about what you eat and not caring too much. It's emotionally and physically healthy to care about eating nutrient-rich foods that make you feel and look good, but it's unhealthy to become so wrapped up in food that it takes away from the rest of your life. The goal isn't to be a perfect eater; again, no such thing

exists! Extremes do not contribute to a healthy life and can even be dangerous. The goal is to be a balanced eater who considers food as just *one* aspect
of health.

Food, of course, serves a pivotal biological function—keeping you alive!
Your body is a machine, and while it can function on low-quality fuel, it
performs at a significantly higher level when you fill it with wholesome,
natural foods. You've probably felt the effects firsthand of eating low-quality
food; after tossing back a sugary donut before an early-morning conference
call, you might feel light-headed, sluggish, and nauseous due to the spike in
blood sugar. It's difficult to concentrate, and your mind keeps wandering off
topic. Maybe the donut constipates you, making your gut feel queasy and
uncomfortable. These horrendous symptoms will likely motivate you to
slam a cup of coffee or eat a second donut just to feel "normal" again for a
few short hours before the cycle begins anew.

The positive effect of quality fuel is just as apparent as the negative
impact of a sugary donut—after eating a bowl of oatmeal topped with a
scoop of peanut butter and a sliced banana for breakfast, you'll feel satisfied
for hours and have the energy to tackle a busy morning. Your mind is sharp
and clear; digestion occurs without bloating or gas; and you don't feel
(super) irritated when your busybody coworker grills you on the latest office
gossip. You might not even need a cup of coffee to wake up. That's because
the oats provide you with whole grains and fiber, the peanut butter delivers
healthy fats and plant protein, and the banana contributes additional natural sugars, vitamins, and minerals. The combination promotes a slower rise
in your blood sugar levels and keeps you sated for hours. All the donut
provides is a shot of processed sugar and flour.

HEALTHIER OATMEAL

Ditch the prepackaged, flavored oatmeal, which is loaded in sugar and artificial flavors. Opt for plain oats and create your own flavors by mixing in different fruits, nuts, and spices. Instructions on how to prepare stovetop and microwaveable oats are on pages 194 and 195.

Food *should* be enjoyed, celebrated, and savored, and yet, at its most basic level, food is fuel for your incredible human machine. Adopting this mentality about what you eat and why can help you take that first step toward reducing the amount of processed food you eat and consuming more wholesome, real foods. If you struggle with honoring your body and respecting its needs, viewing food as fuel is a great way to remove the negative associations you might feel about food. Food as fuel is not code for restriction or missing out on things that taste good! It simply means that, first and foremost, you choose to eat foods that will benefit your overall health instead of foods that simply fill up your belly.

Food as fuel is not about what you'll be taking away, but what you'll be *adding* to your plate. When you think of food as fuel, you look at your plate and think, "Do these foods benefit me nutritionally? What can I add or swap in to this meal to make it healthier for my body?" Fueling well is a reinforcing habit; you'll instantly notice a difference in your energy levels, digestion, and emotions, which will enable you to make better food choices at the next meal.

A Healthy Tipping Point promise—food as fuel does not equal gnawing on cardboard and twigs. Not only will this eating style make you feel healthier and more energetic, it can also taste delicious. Healthy eating does not equal plain or boring!

Healthy Tipping Point Success Story: Tanya, 19, Pennsylvania

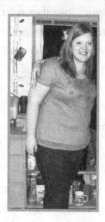 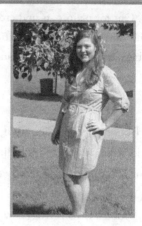

In high school, I was a positive person, participated in an extensive list of extracurricular activities, and was even on the homecoming court. However, when I graduated high school and began college, stress ramped up, and I gained the Freshman 15.

One evening, a group of friends and I met up for an all-night study group. We went on a junk food run to "get us through the long night of studying," and I bought a multiple-serving bag of Chex Mix. I told myself that I would only eat half that night and save the rest for later, but I mindlessly devoured the entire bag while studying. That bag of Chex Mix was my Healthy Tipping Point moment. I looked at the crumbs and knew I needed to make a huge change in my life, once and for all.

Although my life needed a complete overhaul, I decided to focus on changing things step-by-step. I tackled my eating habits first. Even though I was in college and surrounded by processed junk food, I sought out more natural foods like whole grains, tons of produce, lean meats, nuts, and Greek yogurt in the dining hall and the grocery store. After a while, a baked sweet potato and hearty salad with veggies and protein actually sounded better than a greasy pizza.

As my eating habits changed, I realized that I had been using food as a coping mechanism. I would eat when I was bored, upset, or stressed. That's something I continue to struggle with, but I'm implementing more positive coping mechanisms. If I'm stressed and need a mental break, I read a magazine or blog, paint my nails, call my best friend, or go for a walk. I also try to actually think about whatever is stressing me out, instead of just smothering my emotions in food.

I also started to exercise, first by working out on the elliptical machine and later by attending fun workout classes, like the dance class Zumba and spinning, a stationary bike class. Much to my surprise, I discovered that developing an exercise habit was quite easy for me! I realized that working out could be fun—it wasn't at all like my horrific high school gym class! And it's neat to see my fitness extend beyond the gym. When taking the stairs, I used to struggle, but now I can actually sprint from one floor to the next.

People say that they don't have the time to eat well and exercise, but I make time for these healthy habits. You just have to find a way to make it work for you. Eating well and working out triggered a snowball of positivity, encouraging me to get back in the game of life. In a little over half a year, I went from 218 pounds to 153 pounds, losing the Freshman 15 and then some. Although I am still considered medically overweight, I am so much healthier than I used to be, and I'm dedicated to continuing this lifestyle.

Six Healthy Tipping Point Shifts for Healthier Eating

It's fitting that the Standard American Diet's acronym is SAD because the average American's diet is nothing to smile about. In fact, the SAD style of eating is a recipe for disaster. Most Americans (and many other people who live in developed nations) eat a diet that is heavily focused on processed carbohydrates, sodium, and added sugar. In fact, according to the Dietary

Guidelines for Americans, 2010, the top five sources of calories Americans consume come from chicken, bread, pizza, soda and other sweetened beverages, and desserts like cupcakes, pies, and cookies. These foods are filled with little nutrition, low in fiber and whole grains, and packed with calories. Not a single vegetable or fruit made the top five list—none.

SODA'S UNSWEET SIDE

A study by the *American Journal of Public Health* found that people who drink more than two cans of soda a day are three times more likely to be depressed and anxious, compared to those who drink fewer. Soda's sugar and caffeine content, and the resulting impact on your physical health, may be to blame.

Heavy on the sweets, simple carbohydrates, and processed meat, the SAD fills you with low-quality fuel that does nothing for your overall health; in fact, this style of eating is the perfect storm for cancer, heart disease, and digestive disorders. Diseases that many of us accept as a normal part of aging are actually triggered by a lifetime of poor fueling. In striking contrast, people who choose to eat a diet that is the reverse of the SAD have significantly lower incidences of cancer and heart disease. The opposite of SAD is the Healthy Tipping Point style of eating: rich in nutrients; high in fruits and vegetables; high in whole grains and fiber; and low in processed meats and flours, added sodium and sugar, and other fake foods, like artificial sweeteners and flavorings. Simply put, it's a natural, wholesome, nutrient-dense, and *tasty* way to eat.

In one twenty-eight-year study of more than 72,000 women, researchers determined that a diet high in vegetables, fruits, legumes (beans), fish, poultry, and whole grains was associated with a 28 percent lower risk of dying from heart disease than women who regularly consumed meat laden with saturated fat, processed meat (like deli meats, hot dogs, and cured meats), refined grains, French fries, and sweets and desserts. The group who ate in the SAD style also had a 16 percent higher risk of mortality from cancer than women who ate a more "prudent" diet.[9]

What makes a diet healthy or not often boils down to balance. A diet must be able to support your body's short- and long-term physical needs by providing the right amount of energy (calories) and essential nutrients—carbohydrates, proteins, fats, vitamins, minerals, and water—to support your lifestyle. At the same time, a diet is unhealthy if there is too much or too little of a particular nutritional component. This deficiency or excess may increase the risk of developing a chronic disease. (Of course, food is just one part of a complex equation for optimal health; lifestyle choices and genetics matter, too.) If you think about diet on an individual or even on a global basis, it is obvious that the margin for healthy is pretty wide—healthy Americans may eat quite differently from healthy Chinese or healthy Brazilians, but healthy is still healthy.

However, there are some things that all healthy diets have in common: the focus is on real food, specifically minimally processed, plant-based whole foods. Why plants? This topic will be explored throughout the book, but the simple answer is this: plants are nutrient dense but lower in calories when compared to animal products like meat, dairy, and eggs.

The style of eating outlined below is a truly healthy, balanced, and maintainable style of eating that not only tastes good but can actually transform your body to be its leanest and healthiest. If you're in the beginning stages of your healthy journey and gravitate more toward the SAD style of eating, don't feel like you need to do a diet overhaul overnight. "Don't set yourself up to fail; set yourself up for success" is a wonderful healthy living motto that you can adopt for any of your goals, but it is especially applicable to healthy eating. While weight-loss reality television shows often make a dramatic show of cleaning out a contestant's fridge and pantry, tossing all the offending foods into a garbage bag, this just isn't practical for most people! Sudden changes in your eating style might cause you to construct mental roadblocks, such as the dangerous all-or-nothing attitude. The truth is that you don't have to go all the way immediately; making small efforts can really add up.

The suggestions outlined below are described in terms of Healthy Tipping Point shifts for this very reason. Making small shifts in your eating patterns is more maintainable than drastic changes and will still make a tremendous difference in your overall health, especially as each shift builds on another over time. You could start off by making small tweaks to your grocery trips each week; for instance, you could buy whole wheat bread instead of white, or protein-packed, all-natural Greek yogurt instead of artificially sweetened and artificially flavored yogurt. You could also begin by cleaning up one meal, such as breakfast. Or you could vow to pack healthy snacks to take to work so you're not stuck dropping quarters into the vending machine for a sugary three o'clock pick-me-up.

Advice on healthy eating can get a little complicated—What are omega-3s and what exactly do they do? What the heck is a flexitarian? Should I buy fat-free dairy products?—so let's boil down the information you're about to digest. The six Healthy Tipping Point shifts for healthier eating are changes:

- To real food
- To plant-focused foods
- To whole grains
- To trans-fat-free foods
- To fiber
- To balance

FLEXITARIANISM

Flexitarianism is a fun way to describe an eating style that is strongly focused on plants but does not restrict animal products. A flexitarian eats mainly plant-based protein and meatless meals but occasionally enjoys meat or fish. This no-rules approach to eating encourages a healthy and balanced plant-packed diet that the majority of people can easily integrate into their lifestyle.

To Real Food

With all the startling data about the negative effects of the SAD, it's not surprising that terms like "processed food" and "unprocessed food" are quickly becoming media buzzwords. However, the term "processed" can be confusing. If a processed food is a food that has been altered from its natural state, isn't cheese processed because it's pasteurized? What about fruit juice? Or frozen veggies? Does this mean these products are inherently worse for you than their cleaner cousins: raw cheese, whole fruit, and fresh veggies? Not necessarily! It's enough to make my head spin—and probably yours, too.

> If you can't pronounce it, think twice about eating it.

An easier way to think about this issue is in terms of real food versus fake food. Real food tends to have a very short ingredients list—maybe just one ingredient! Fake food, or food made from ingredients created in a laboratory, has a much, much longer ingredients list, including artificial food additives and preservatives. The fake food is then "enriched" by adding back the vitamins stripped away during processing or "fortified" by adding nutrients that were never in the food in the first place—like adding vitamins to candy. Food producers aren't doing this solely for the benefit of your health; it's also a sneaky marketing ploy to give fake foods a healthy halo, which lures consumers. Don't buy into the marketing on the front of the box. Read the ingredients list and ask yourself, "Is this a real food or a fake food?"

The Food and Drug Administration (FDA) oversees the approval of all food additives; unfortunately, the agency has bowed to industry pressures in the past, green-lighting additives that were deemed potentially harmful to animal and human health during laboratory testing. The FDA typically approves these questionable additives because research shows they are only harmful in massive quantities. When it comes to our health, is it sensible for the FDA to take such a relaxed approach? I vote no!

REAL FOOD AT THE GROCERY STORE

Keep it simple at the grocery store—don't go up and down every aisle. Most of the real food is located around the perimeter of the store. Much of the food on the inner shelves includes extra salt and preservatives to extend shelf life. Several notable exceptions to the perimeter rule include whole grains, like brown rice or oatmeal, canned low-sodium beans, and frozen plain fruits or vegetables. Frozen produce is nutritionally similar to fresh produce because the fruits and veggies are picked at their peak freshness, and their nutrition is locked in when the produce is flash-frozen at the processing plant.

Our society has become so accustomed to consuming fake foods that most of us don't bat an eye when we pick up yogurt with ingredients like gelatin, potassium sorbate, and carmine—mostly because we have no idea what these things are or do! Gelatin is a gelling agent derived from animal skin and bones, potassium sorbate is a food preservative, and carmine is a food coloring derived from crushed insects. Yes, really. To make matters worse, these are the ingredients in a popular *children's* yogurt. Real yogurt requires only two ingredients, milk and cultured bacteria, not ten.

While some fake-food ingredients are questionable (does anyone really want to eat crushed beetles in their yogurt?), other additives are just outright dangerous—but that doesn't mean they are illegal. Certain common food additives, which are listed in the table below, have been shown to contribute to cancer, behavioral problems, heart disease, and allergic reactions. Even though these ingredients are suspect, they are still on the market and in the foods we eat. Most people believe the government—the Food and Drug Administration, specifically—regulates ingredients to ensure this type of thing doesn't happen. While the FDA has banned many harmful ingredients, other countries, especially those in the European Union, take a much more prudent approach and have outlawed many more additives. For example, the EU has banned many artificial food dyes; European food manufacturers use natural coloring, like strawberries and beets, to give their foods a red hue. In America, we still use a dye created in a laboratory—Red 40.

It's important to note that not all scary-sounding fake-food ingredients are necessarily bad for you. For example, maltodextrin is a thickener, filler, or binding agent made from rice, corn, or potato starch. Yes, it's created in a laboratory, and yes, it's processed; however, consuming food additives like maltodextrin is certainly nothing to worry about.

There are literally hundreds of food additives out there, and it can be difficult to remember which may be potentially dangerous and which are safe to consume. The table below lists eleven food additives that everyone should avoid, according to the Center for Science in the Public Interest, a nonprofit consumer advocacy group focused on nutritional education. The CSPI's Web site also lists additives that should be consumed only in small amounts, as well as additives that certain people, like pregnant women or people who are allergic to gluten, should avoid. These additives include Blue 1, Red 40, carmine, casein, hydrolyzed vegetable protein, and monosodium glutamate (MSG).

ELEVEN FOOD ADDITIVES TO AVOID

Additive	Common Sources	Reason to Avoid
Acesulfame-K or Acesulfame	This additive is an artificial sweetener that is often found in baked goods, chewing gum, diet sodas, and gel-based desserts.	Like many artificial sweeteners, the jury is still out on acesulfame-K; however, some studies have linked the sweetener to cancer and thyroid issues.
Artificial colorings (specifically, Blue 2, Red 3, Yellow 5, and Yellow 6)	Artificial colorings are found in a variety of packaged foods, including beverages, candies, cereals, and more.	Although the FDA has concluded that each of these colorings is safe for consumption, animal studies have tentatively linked them to cancer, tumors, and other health problems, including allergic reactions and hyperactivity in children.
Aspartame (Equal, NutraSweet)	Like acesulfame-K, aspartame is an artificial sweetener and is found in similar products.	Although data has been inconclusive, evidence exists that excessive consumption of aspartame, especially from a young age, increases cancer risk.
Butylated hydroxyanisole (BHA)	BHA prevents packaged foods that contain oil and fat from going rancid on the shelf. It is often found in cereal, potato chips, and vegetable oil. BHA can also be found in pet food and in cosmetics and other nonfood products.	Some evidence suggests that BHA may cause cancer in the forestomach of rats, mice, and hamsters. Even though humans do not have forestomachs, the U.S. Department of Health and Human Services has stated that BHA is "reasonably anticipated to be a human carcinogen." Despite these findings, the FDA still permits it to be used in foods.
Caramel coloring	Caramel coloring gives food products a deep, rich coloring and is often used in baked goods, gravy, precooked meats, and soda.	Caramel coloring is the most commonly added coloring by weight to food products, which is one of the reasons it should be avoided. Caramel coloring contains 2-methylimidazole and 4-methylimidazole, two contaminants that have been identified as possible carcinogens.

Additive	Common Sources	Reason to Avoid
Olestra (Olean)	Olestra is a fat substitute used in some potato chips.	Olestra is a synthetic fat that cannot be absorbed by the digestive system, which makes it zero calories. Eating too much olestra at a time can result in unexpected diarrhea, cramping, and gas. The fat also temporarily inhibits the absorption of some nutrients from vegetables and fruits.
Partially hydrogenated vegetable oil	Also known as trans fat, partially hydrogenated vegetable oil is used in margarine, fried foods, microwave popcorn, baked goods, and other packaged foods.	Partially hydrogenated vegetable oil has been linked to heart disease and other health issues. A more complete review of trans fat is provided later in this chapter.
Potassium bromate	Potassium bromote increases the volume of white flour when baked and can be found in bread and rolls.	This additive usually breaks down to form the harmless potassium bromide; however, trace amounts of potassium bromate may be found in the finished bread product. Potassium bromate has been linked to cancer in animals.
Propyl gallate	This additive is a preservative used in vegetable oil, meat products, chicken soups, and chewing gum.	Laboratory analyses have inconclusively linked propyl gallate to cancer in animals.
Saccharin (Sweet'N Low)	Saccharin is an artificial sweetener commonly used in diet soda and no-sugar-added products.	Many studies have strongly linked saccharin to bladder cancer in animals; further studies have shown a link between saccharin and other types of cancer as well. Food products containing saccharin were previously required to include a warning label about its ill effects; however, Congress removed this requirement in 2000, partly in response to pressures from the diet-food industry.

Additive	Common Sources	Reason to Avoid
Sodium nitrate / Sodium nitrite	This additive blocks the growth of bacteria in cured meats. It also gives cured meat a red color. Without it, hot dogs and bacon would appear gray. This may be one of the major reasons manufacturers push to keep it legalized. Sodium nitrate and sodium nitrite can also be found in many deli meats, breakfast sausages, meat jerkies, and meat-based canned soups.	When added to food, sodium nitrate and sodium nitrite can lead to the formation of nitrosamines, a cancer-causing chemical. Manufacturers often add ascorbic acid or erythorbic acid to hamper this reaction; however, these additives do not eliminate the risks associated with sodium nitrate and sodium nitrite.

Source: "Chemical Cuisine" from the Center for Science in the Public Interest, 2011.

One thing you might notice when reading over the eleven food additives to avoid is that all of these potentially dangerous food additives are found mainly in SAD packaged foods, especially meats and sweets. Thus, by reducing our consumption of packaged foods, we automatically reduce the amount of food additives we're ingesting.

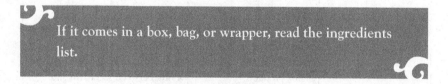

If it comes in a box, bag, or wrapper, read the ingredients list.

Another easy way to reduce your dependency on fake foods is to remember the Less Boxes guideline. Fake food is, inherently, packaged in boxes and bags. The Less Boxes guideline is a great visual trick to use when you're at the grocery store—look down into your cart and see how many colorful boxes you've got in there. Many real foods—like fruits and veggies—don't have any packaging at all (of course, some real food, like rice, must be packaged). The fewer boxes you have in the cart, the more real food you are probably eating.

Humans have made incredible advancements in science and technology; however, perhaps food is one thing that shouldn't be tinkered with. Most packaged foods shout out snazzy marketing catchphrases—"Now with added fiber to promote digestion!" or "Fortified with vitamins and minerals!" Each of these claims signals that something has been added to the food unnaturally, making it more fake food than real food. In reality, these "added-to" foods contain nothing you couldn't get from eating a well-rounded real-food diet. Food fads come and go—scientists claimed margarine was a healthy alternative to butter until they realized the devastating impact of trans fat on the cardiovascular system! What is deemed safe now might be labeled unhealthy in ten years' time.

The Healthy Tipping Point shift away from processed and packaged foods to unprocessed or minimally processed real foods is the surest, simplest way to achieve long-term health. Real food is never a fad!

To Plant-Focused Foods

Americans are obsessed with meat. Our meals revolve around meat, poultry, fish, and other animal products, such as dairy and eggs. When we plan our dishes, animal flesh is often the focus of the meal. Most of us skimp on or entirely skip the vegetables. Grains are usually processed, not whole grain, and take up a fair share of the plate. On average, we eat eight ounces of meat a day (twice the global average), and to feed this demand, our farmers slaughter ten *billion* animals a year.

NO PRESSURE

Protein is an essential part of your diet, but protein doesn't have to come just from animal meat—plants have protein, too. And a plant-based diet doesn't mean you have to forgo meat, poultry, or fish if you don't want to; it's about simply eating *more plants*. Don't read "plant-based diet" and feel pressured to give anything up. This way of eating is merely about filling your plate with more plants: whole grains, seeds, nuts, vegetables, or fruits. Remember—your body, your diet, your rules.

The reasons behind our excessive animal-product consumption are complex. We've been culturally conditioned to enjoy the taste and associate it with wealth, happiness, and abundance (Thanksgiving turkey is a perfect example). Meat is perceived as inexpensive and convenient, but plant proteins, like beans, are actually much cheaper. Furthermore, the vast majority of the meat industry seeks to keep the cost of meats as low as possible by feeding most of the animals cheap grains instead of a more natural diet of grass; dosing animals with large amounts of antibiotics, hormones, and other medications; and raising them in less-than-ideal and tightly packed conditions. Many people believe that eating animal protein and large amounts of dairy is *necessary*, not just for weight loss, bone density, or muscle development, but for basic functioning. We've been led to believe that animal protein is an irreplaceable component to a healthy diet. And yet this couldn't be further from the truth.

Let's be clear: this shift is not about restriction. This shift is about *adding* something to your diet—the healthy and nutritional goodness plants offer in abundance. Shifting toward a plant-based diet does not mean you must become a vegetarian or give up meat or other animal products entirely. The Healthy Tipping Point version of health, as you are undoubtedly beginning to understand, is about creating balance, not stripping it away. Most

Americans completely lack balance when it comes to meat consumption; an excessive amount of animal flesh a day is not balanced! Meat (as well as sweets and processed carbohydrates) have pushed our everyday green friends off our plates. There are many, many reasons to eat *less* meat—the environmental and ethical consequences of such mass production will be explored later in this chapter—but for now, let's focus on the most personally important reason to eat *more* plants: your health.

We consider obesity, cancer, heart disease, diabetes, and other chronic diseases a normal part of the aging process. And yet these diseases have been clearly and inextricably linked to the foods that we eat every day. A juicy cheeseburger and French fries might look and smell appealing, but that meal unleashes a tiny terror in your body, triggering a rise of cholesterol in the bloodstream, a buildup of plaque in the arteries, the modification of important digestive enzymes, an increase in inflammation and cell proliferation, and the development of an acidic environment. Repeat this meal over and over for decades, combine it with the "wrong" genetics, and you have the perfect breeding ground for heart disease and cancer.

Michael Pollan, America's renowned food journalist and a staunch omnivore (eater of everything!), summed up his solution to our national health crisis in eight concise words: "Eat real food, not too much, mostly plants." The health benefits of eating mostly plants cannot be underestimated. Nutrient-dense fruits and vegetables provide the human body with high-quality fuel that helps your body perform efficiently and ward off acute and chronic diseases. In fact, a plant-based diet is the single most effective way to prevent or stop the progression of coronary artery disease, the leading cause of death in the United States, because less animal protein or animal products means less cholesterol and saturated fat.

EAT YOUR WAY TO HEALTH

Diet and other lifestyle choices contribute to approximately 80 percent of colon, breast, and prostate cancer cases and 33 percent of all other types of cancer. People who eat the most vegetables are 50 percent less likely to get cancer than those who eat the least. Your momma was right. Eat your vegetables![10]

Eating a varied plant-based diet is like wearing a coat of armor. Plants fight off heart disease and cancer by neutralizing free radicals (molecules that damage body cells). As you might recall from high school chemistry, an atom or molecule with an unpaired electron is highly reactive. Free radicals are like preschoolers who don't know how to share—they "steal" electrons from nearby stable molecules, creating a new free radical, which attacks the next stable molecule. If left unchecked, free radicals can proliferate and create cell and tissue damage. Antioxidants, which are found in fruits and vegetables, are special molecules that can share their electrons without becoming free radicals themselves, thereby stopping the free-radical cycle in its tracks. Plants have other important qualities—fiber, vitamins, and minerals—that also contribute toward greater health and disease prevention.

Quick veggie fix: serve rice or pasta on a bed of raw baby spinach.

Beyond the long-term health benefits, plant-based diets make it easier to reach or maintain a healthy weight. When you relegate fruits and vegetables to side-dish status, you fill up on calorie-dense carbohydrates and meats. Eating a greater percentage of fruits and vegetables can reduce your overall caloric intake, which may help you reach or maintain a healthy weight. For example, if you swapped a five-inch piece of buttered garlic bread for a cup of the Simple Roasted Broccoli (page 225), you'd save hundreds of calories and add tons of nutritional value to your meal. Thanks to the boost of fiber, you'd also feel fuller for longer despite the calorie reduction.

There's another surprising benefit to cutting back on your meat consumption: it's economical! In a world of one-dollar cheeseburgers and ninety-nine-cent ground-beef tacos, a plant-based diet sounds fancy and expensive. In reality, vegetarian protein staples (beans, lentils, tofu) are significantly cheaper than quality meat alternatives. Eating less meat will slash your grocery bills.

On that note, here's a quick word about faux meat products: they can be very pricey (vegetarian sausage, for example, runs about five dollars for five sausages). While such imitation meat products can help many people wean off of entirely meat-centered diets, they often contain loads of fake-food ingredients and are often high in sodium. Furthermore, research suggests that eating too much processed soy—especially soy protein isolate—may be harmful, so these meat alternatives should be consumed in moderation, if at all.

As you move away from eating processed foods and toward unprocessed, natural foods, you will undoubtedly begin to eat a diet that is richer in plants. This shift is all about bringing these plants to center stage. So much of this shift is about proportions; meat and other animal products do not need to be the focus of your meals. A healthier diet is one that is centered on vegetables, fruits, beans, nuts, whole grains, and plant protein sources. If you're not ready to go *meatless*, make it your goal to simply eat *less meat*. In this scenario, less really is more. Make room for the plants!

FIVE WAYS TO PAINLESSLY REDUCE YOUR ANIMAL PRODUCT CONSUMPTION

1. Swap deli meat for nut butters, beans, or hummus (check out the Spinach Hummus recipe on page 231).
2. Explore different cuisines. Indian and Thai restaurants offer a wide range of meat-free dishes like vegetable korma, tofu pad thai, and panang curry.
3. Swap cow's milk for unsweetened soy or hemp milk (for concerns about calcium in nondairy alternatives, flip to page 141). Other milk alternatives include almond or rice milk, but these alternatives don't offer much protein.
4. Try vegetarian sushi. Many Japanese restaurants will craft a fish-free roll from avocado, carrots, beets, tofu, cucumbers, asparagus, or zucchini.
5. Top salads with chickpeas instead of chicken. To reduce sodium by nearly half, drain and rinse the beans first.

Healthy Tipping Point Success Story:
Shelley, 24, Colorado

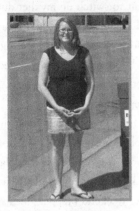 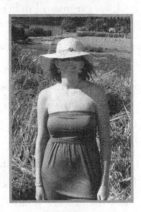

I used to eat the traditional Southerner's diet—roasts, fried chicken, fried fish, burgers, and anything and everything creamy or cheesy. Even my green beans were cooked in bacon grease! I really never thought about what I ate or why, but looking back, there was a lot more going on than just Southern cookin'. I would eat when I was sad, happy, bored, or struggling with low self-esteem. Emotional eating only made me feel worse and guilty, and then I would eat more. At just twenty-three, I found myself unhappy and overweight. I knew I needed to change.

Then, several things happened at once: I graduated college and moved to Colorado—there are so many fun and healthy outdoor activities here! I loved the experience of hiking; however, I couldn't finish a trail . . . I simply wasn't fit enough. This only motivated me to work harder. I was sick of feeling tired, sluggish, and depressed. Around the same time, I got engaged, and I really wanted to feel good on the inside and look good on the outside on my wedding day.

One day, I was flipping through a magazine when a recipe caught my eye: stuffed squash, a vegan alternative to the traditional Thanksgiving turkey. I said to my fiancé, "If more vegetarian food looked like this, then I would have no problem eating that way all the time!" I ordered a bunch of cookbooks by the recipe's author, Nava Atlas, with the premise of getting more veggies in my diet. I was planning to do a one-week vegan experiment when I found out I was pregnant. I didn't want to switch up my diet during my pregnancy, so I continued to eat a flexitarian diet—but then I miscarried several weeks into the pregnancy while my husband was serving in Afghanistan. Feeling completely alone and down in the dumps, I decided to try a week of veganism to give me something positive to focus on. I felt so amazing at the end of the week that I kept it up.

My favorite snacks are apples, bananas, or rice cakes with smears of peanut butter. I also really enjoy a simple bowl of cereal with ice-cold almond milk. I've even started baking vegan desserts, like chocolate chip cookies! I've found that preparation is key for making a plant-based diet work. I usually spend a few hours on the weekend prepping meals for the upcoming workweek; for example, I blend and freeze smoothies, wash and cut veggies, and boil and refrigerate rice. This makes it easier to create healthy meals during the workweek.

A year and a half after starting my healthy living journey and transitioning to a plant-based diet, I am down fifty pounds and filled with confidence, happiness, and self-love. Because I put more thought into what I eat and why, I feel so much more connected to the natural world around me. I've even encouraged my friends and family to be healthier in their own ways, too. My husband even eats more plants than he did before, even though he didn't go all the way to a vegan diet with me.

To Whole Grains

There's no reason to fear carbohydrates—they're essential to your very existence, and carbs are a pivotal source of energy for your body. In fact, your brain runs exclusively on carbohydrates in the form of glucose. The trouble with carbs is that many people eat too many refined carbohydrates, which are processed and usually have fewer nutrients compared to unrefined carbohydrates. Refined carbohydrates, including sweetened drinks, desserts, and even some "healthy" granola, are often packed with added sugar. Consuming refined carbohydrates, especially when you eat too many refined carbs and not enough protein or fat in the same meal or snack, leads to what is commonly referred to as a sugar surge and crash.

As the sugar floods your bloodstream, your pancreas responds by producing a large amount of insulin, which carries the sugar to your body's cells to store it for later use. The physical crash occurs because the insulin has done such an effective job squirreling away this sugar. Your muscles and brain need some sugar to function, so you'll crave even more sweets, triggering the cycle all over again.

You can avoid this surge-and-crash sensation by opting for a proper serving of carbohydrates from whole grains, which will initiate a much slower, more manageable release of insulin. Whole grains are healthier than refined grains for all the reasons real foods are healthier than fake foods. By simply shifting your diet to include more whole grains instead of refined grains, you'll receive extra fiber and more naturally occurring nutrients. Due to their fiber content, whole grains will also sate your appetite. Best of all, whole grains won't result in any headache-inducing sugar crashes; research indicates that complex carbohydrates enter the bloodstream much more gradually than refined carbs.

WHOLE-GRAIN CODE

Food labels can be tricky—the front of a package will scream, "Multigrain goodness!" but when you read the label, you discover that "multigrain" merely signifies a combination of whole and enriched flours. Brown rice, buckwheat, bulgur, cracked wheat, millet, oats, oatmeal, quinoa, wheat berries, whole-grain barley, whole-grain corn, whole rye, whole spelt, whole wheat, and wild rice are all whole grains. However, the following grains are *not* considered whole grains: bran, corn flour, cornmeal, enriched flour, multigrain, pumpernickel, rice, rice flour, rye flour, stone-ground wheat, wheat, wheat flour, wheat germ, or unbleached wheat flour.

It can be difficult to remember which grains are whole and which are not. In a pinch, just keep your eyes peeled for the word "whole"—if you don't see it, odds are the grain isn't whole. And be sure to read the *entire* ingredients list; often a product's first ingredient will be a whole grain but the next two will be refined grains.

To Trans-Fat-Free Foods

There are three types of fats in foods: unsaturated fats, saturated fats, and trans fats. The one fat you absolutely want to avoid, even in small doses, is trans fat. Trans fat is usually created through a chemical process known as hydrogenation, which makes an unsaturated fat solid at room temperature. The result is a fat that raises LDL levels ("bad" cholesterol) and lowers HDL levels ("good" cholesterol), thus increasing the risk of coronary heart disease, even when trans fat is consumed in very small amounts. Trans fat has also been loosely linked to infertility, poor liver function, depression, and a variety of other health issues.

TRANS FAT FREE . . . EXCEPT WHEN IT'S NOT

Trans fat is present in many store-bought baked goods, crackers, and cookies because it increases shelf life and is cheaper than using other types of fats. Trans fat might also be found in fried foods. Under current FDA regulations, manufacturers can claim the product has zero grams of trans fat if the serving contains less than 0.5 grams of trans fat. If that sounds ridiculous, that's because it is *completely* ridiculous—zero should be zero! To ensure you stay trans fat free, scan the ingredients list and avoid any products with the words "shortening," "partially hydrogenated vegetable oil," or "hydrogenated vegetable oil," since these are code words for trans fat.

Saturated fats are linked to rises in LDL cholesterol and are found in animal products, including meat and dairy, as well as in tropical oils. Although saturated fats, like butter or coconut oil, work well for cooking, saturated fats should be consumed in moderation. Unsaturated fats are a tasty *and* healthy alternative to saturated fat. Unsaturated fats are typically from plant sources; studies have indicated unsaturated fats increase HDL cholesterol.

Olive oil, canola oil, avocados, peanut oils, peanuts, and cashews contain monounsaturated fats, thought to be the healthiest type of unsaturated fats. Each of these oils has its own distinctly different taste and cooks best under different conditions. Extra-virgin olive oil makes the tastiest dressings, and virgin olive oil works well in stir-fries. Canola oil, on the other hand, has a higher smoke point (when the oil begins to burn) and should be used for high-heat cooking, like baking or roasting.

To Fiber

When you make the shifts toward whole grains and toward more fruits and veggies, you'll have this shift covered—but the importance of fiber cannot be underestimated! After all, regularly eating an adequate amount of fiber improves cholesterol levels, reduces blood pressure, decreases inflammation, and stabilizes blood sugar levels. It is thought that fiber can also bind to many toxins, moving them out of the body faster. Fiber can also be credited with weight maintenance, since consuming fiber contributes to a feeling of fullness without adding calories.

Our bodies need two types of fiber for optimal health: soluble fiber and insoluble fiber. Whole fruits and vegetables are great sources of both kinds.

Other sources of soluble fiber include nuts, oats, bran, and beans; insoluble fiber sources include whole-grain products (cereals, pasta, bread) and bran.

> On Monday, bring five pieces of fresh fruit to work and store them in a basket on your desk. Snack on one every afternoon.

Soluble fiber absorbs water and combines with the food in your small intestine to form a thick gel. This allows the nutrients in the food you eat to be absorbed gradually during the digestion process; this is especially important to stabilize blood sugar levels. The gel mixture also holds on to the cholesterol added to the mix by digestive bile and prevents it from being reabsorbed into your blood, thereby reducing blood cholesterol levels. Soluble fiber is also important because it adds water to your stools, keeping you from becoming constipated, and serves as "food" (prebiotics) for all the friendly digestive bacteria in your colon.

Insoluble fiber simply moves through your digestive track unchanged, taking up space (and therefore reducing appetite). It also bulks up your stools, thereby creating a need to "go" more regularly, which is excellent for digestive health. In addition, insoluble fiber can reduce symptoms of irritable bowel syndrome, prevent hemorrhoids and diverticulosis, and may also help prevent colon cancer

Women should eat twenty-five grams of fiber a day (men need about thirty-five grams), which is roughly the amount of fiber in five servings of fruits and vegetables and one to two servings of whole grains or beans. If you're eating the clean, real-food diet advocated in this book, you're probably meeting or exceeding your daily fiber needs.

FULL OF FIBER

Adding fiber to your diet too quickly can feel like a party is going down in your gut. If you experience excessive gas, bloating, and abdominal pain, reduce the amount of fiber-rich foods you're consuming to a comfortable level. Add back five grams of fiber a day, allowing a week before another five-gram increase. It's also important to drink a lot of water while increasing the fiber in your diet. Fiber needs water to pass through your system easily; without it, constipation results.

And yes—you can eat too much fiber, even if your gut can handle it. More than thirty-five grams a day can push food through your intestines so quickly that your body doesn't have an opportunity to fully absorb important nutrients. Too much fiber can also trigger painful constipation. Be mindful of fake foods with inulin, a soluble added fiber used in certain breads, granola bars, and yogurts. While it's fine to eat a little inulin, it can easily add up and back *you* up. If you eat enough veggies and fruits, you don't need products with extra fiber.

To Balance

When it comes to eating in balance, there are three important aspects to consider: serving sizes, the frequency of so-called discretionary foods, and the timing and size of meals.

Serving Sizes

The old expression "feast with your eyes" could not be more true. In fact, your brain relies mostly on visual cues—not how full your stomach feels—to determine if you are sated. Before we even take a bite, most people use their eyes to assess how much food they intend to eat and will eat to that point, regardless of whether they are full before the predetermined point. In fact, 54 percent of Americans claim they usually eat until their plate is clean. The trouble with this visual dining is that portion sizes continue to increase steadily, in restaurants and at home, so people are inadvertently eating more and more.

For example, twenty years ago, a restaurant portion of spaghetti with meatballs equaled 500 calories (or one cup of spaghetti with sauce and three meatballs). Now, the average portion of spaghetti and meatballs equals 1,025 calories (or two cups of spaghetti with sauce and three large meatballs). No matter how hungry, most diners will eat the entire portion of spaghetti and meatballs simply because that's what is served to them.

In a 2004 study, researchers decided to put the visual dining research to the test in a very sneaky way. A restaurant table was rigged so that researchers could slowly refill the soup bowls through a tube as the participant ate. These "never-ending" bowls of soup tested whether participants relied on visual cues (an empty bowl) or satiety cues to determine whether they were full.

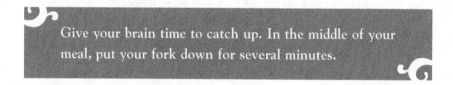

Give your brain time to catch up. In the middle of your meal, put your fork down for several minutes.

Amazingly, participants who ate from the never-ending bowl consumed 73 percent more; despite the extra food, they did not rate themselves as any more full than the participants who ate from the regular bowls!

The research on visual dining is clear: we can't necessarily rely on a cursory glance at our food to determine how much of it we should be eating, especially when we're eating from a multiple-serving bag or box (like chips or cookies) or out at a restaurant. A portion, which is how much we eat at one time, is different from a serving, which is the standard unit of measuring food (usually by cups or ounces). A giant muffin from a coffee shop might be eaten in one portion, but it's usually two servings, for example. Keeping portions under control is an easy way to clean up your diet and ensure you're not overeating.

The most important tool for portion control is right at your fingertips: the nutrition label. A packaged food always comes with a nutrition label; real food (like fruits and veggies) often don't have packages with labels, but you can look up the nutritional information online. Most chain restaurants also provide nutritional information online.

Provided below is a nutrition label for a popular brand of trail mix that contains peanuts, raisins, chocolate pieces, almonds, and cashews.

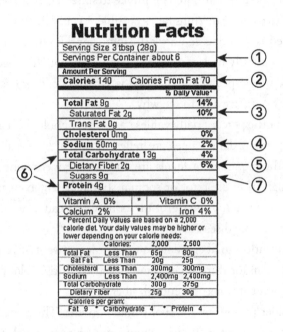

When reading a nutrition label, you'll want to take note of the following things:

1. Compare the serving size to the number of servings per container. Many people assume the nutrition label is for the entire package, but that's not always the case. This label, for example, provides the data for one-sixth of the bag.

2. The next important bit of information on the label is the calories and calories from fat per serving. More information on calories and

how your caloric intake impacts a healthy lifestyle is provided on page 122. Remember that the calorie count is for one serving; in this example, a serving of trail mix has 140 calories, but the entire bag has 840 (140 calories times six servings).

3. Check out the types of fat present in the food. Dietary fat is not a bad thing; in fact, it's absolutely essential to life! But you don't want to overeat saturated fats (the American Heart Association recommends you limit saturated fat intake to sixteen grams a day), and you want to eat as little trans fat as possible. Even if the trans fat content is listed as zero, double-check the ingredients for words like "shortening," "partially hydrogenated vegetable oil," or "hydrogenated vegetable oil," especially if the food is a baked good or packaged treat (check out page 110 to see why).

4. Look at the percent daily values (% DV) for cholesterol and sodium. The percent daily values are reflections of a 2,000-calorie-per-day diet; the requirement levels are set by the government. Foods that are high in cholesterol or sodium should be eaten in moderation, since too much cholesterol or sodium can cause or contribute to many chronic diseases.

5. Pay attention to fiber. Women need at least twenty-five grams; men should aim for thirty-five grams. If you're eating a plant-based diet, you're probably getting enough fiber.

6. Consider protein and carbohydrate content. The Healthy Tipping Point style of eating is more about balancing your meals than strictly counting macronutrients like carbohydrates, protein, or fat; it's a good idea to know what's in the foods you're eating and plan when you are going to eat them. For example, a carb-rich snack is the ideal preworkout fuel, and a food with more protein is better to eat after a hard workout (to see why, refer to The Best Pre- and Postworkout Fuel on page 256).

7. Shake down the sugar. The sugar entry on the nutrition label can be especially helpful if you're torn between two similar products, like cereal or granola bars, and want to compare the amount of sugar. (Just

read the ingredients list to ensure there are no artificial sweeteners in the mix.) But although a nutrition label tells you how many grams of sugar are in the food, it doesn't tell you where it comes from. Orange juice, for example, has about twenty-one grams of sugar per serving, but that's all from the sugars that naturally occur in fruit. Cereal, on the other hand, can have just as much sugar, but it's *added* sugars.

8. Last, size up the ingredients list. Usually located below the nutrition label, the ingredients list will tell you whether the food is primarily comprised of real food or fake food. The ingredients list might also explain some of the nutrition facts; if a slice of cake seems too low in calories to be true, it might be packed with artificial sweeteners instead of real sugar.

SAFE SWEETENERS

Although many people are hesitant to eat foods with added sugar, consider this—a little bit of real sugar is much healthier than a bunch of artificial sweeteners (if you have a medical condition that requires you to limit your sugar intake, ask your doctor for their opinion). One tablespoon of real sugar adds a mere 45 calories to your coffee, and it's way tastier than artificial sweeteners such as acesulfame-K, aspartame, and saccharin.

Natural alternatives include agave nectar, honey, and stevia. Agave nectar and honey pack a sweet punch, so you don't need to use a lot. Stevia, which is derived from a plant, is a tasty no-calorie sweetener; however, long-term research on stevia is limited, and it would be wise to eat it in moderation until more is known.

While reading and analyzing the nutrition label might seem tedious, you'll learn to absorb the most significant information with a quick glance. Perhaps it is most important to simply familiarize yourself with normal serving sizes for your favorite foods. And don't worry—you don't need to carry a measuring cup around all the time to ensure you're eating the right amount. Portion control can be easy if you follow these simple tips:

- Figure out what the serving sizes of foods you commonly eat actually look like on your plates and in your bowls. Measuring out a cup of cereal just one time, for example, will illustrate whether you should fill your favorite bowl halfway or all the way to the brim.
- When eating at home, serve yourself one portion and place any left-overs in the fridge. If you're tempted for seconds or thirds, wait ten minutes to see if you're still hungry or if you're just riding the momentum of eating.
- On average, if you're like most people, the larger the package, the more you'll eat from it. Try to avoid "multitasking" while eating and eat your food at a table. If you snack at all in front of the television or computer, put the amount you plan to eat on a plate. Eating directly out of the package messes with your ability to assess your satiety.
- If you frequently overeat a particular snack like nuts or trail mix, separate the contents into correct serving sizes and place them in separate plastic bags. Do this when you first open the package.
- Most chain restaurants post nutritional information on their Web sites. Checking out your options beforehand—and noting the serving sizes—will help you make healthier decisions when the waiter asks for your order.
- If you struggle not to eat whatever is on your plate, ask for a to-go box when your food arrives. Immediately box up half of it. Alternatively, split meals with your dining companion.
- Take the time to become familiar with your hunger and sated cues. Instead of wolfing down your food, slow down and enjoy what you're eating. Recognizing when you're full or if you're still hungry goes a long way to reaching and maintaining a healthy weight.

PORTION CONTROL VISUAL GUIDES

Food	Visual Guide
One serving of a fruit or vegetable	Baseball
One serving of ice cream	Tennis ball
One serving of nuts	Golf ball
One serving of meat or chicken	Deck of cards
One serving of fish	An iPhone
One serving of cereal	Two hands cupped together
One serving of peanut butter	Golf ball
One serving of pasta	Tennis ball
One serving of cheese	Four dice
One serving of grains (rice or quinoa, for example)	Baseball

Discretionary Foods

The Healthy Tipping Point style of eating says you can eat anything you want—as long as you do it in balance with the rest of your diet. Do you want some chocolate cake? Eat a slice! But eat a moderate slice, not half the cake, and savor each bite. Moderation applies to more than serving size; moderation also refers to frequency. Do you want French fries? Eat some fries! Just don't eat fries every single day; make them a once-in-a-while treat.

Foods like chocolate cake and French fries are discretionary foods, or foods that you elect to eat simply because they taste good, not necessarily for any particular health benefit. Some people refer to discretionary foods as treats, splurges, or indulgences—"I'm going to be 'bad' and eat these onion rings," they'll say. But these names cast discretionary foods in an inherently negative light. There's nothing wrong with eating dessert or potato chips—trust me! The trouble comes with overdoing it and eating these foods too often or in extra-large portions.

It's completely fine to enjoy a small portion of discretionary food—a half cup of ice cream or a fun-sized candy bar—every day. Or you can save up your discretionary food and eat a larger serving of your favorite foods once or twice a week, if you wish. Enjoying discretionary foods is part of life, and there's absolutely no reason why you can't eat your favorite foods in moderation and in balance with the rest of your diet.

> Keep cookies and baked goods in the freezer, not the pantry; you'll be less tempted to mindlessly munch.

Portion control of discretionary foods can be difficult if you struggle with emotional eating. If you feel an urge to continue eating after you've had a proper portion of food, take a break from the table. Change the scenery and focus your mind on another task—go for a walk, tidy up your bedroom, call a friend, or check your e-mails. I find that making a cup of tea is particularly effective because it gives my hands, mind, and taste buds something to focus on. Give your brain some breathing space and then reassess whether you really want to go back for more food. If your urge to eat is more emotional than physical, the desire to continue eating may pass naturally once you move on to other things.

If you're still physically hungry after waiting fifteen minutes, have a bit more food. When your body presents signs of hunger (growling stomach or light-headedness, for example), you should always eat, even if it's not on schedule or you feel that your last meal should have satisfied you. After all, your caloric needs vary from day to day, and you shouldn't fight biology.

It is often helpful to remember that *the treats will be there tomorrow.* So often, we overeat goodies because we feel like if we don't eat them, we'll miss out. Maybe that's true on Thanksgiving—when else do you get pumpkin pie?!—but it's certainly not true for store-bought cookies or office birthday cake. There's no reason to go overboard and throw portion control out the window when the foods will always be available.

Timing and Size of Meals

The final aspect of balanced eating relates to the sizing and timing of your meals. Many SAD eaters skip breakfast and eat an oversize dinner. This wreaks havoc on your system. After all, by the time you wake up, you've gone at least eight hours without food, maybe longer. If you wait until lunch to eat, you're nearing fourteen hours without food. At this point, your body is literally running on fumes.

If you eat most of your calories at night, your body must work overtime to digest the meal when it should, ideally, be resting. Not only that, but anything it digests and can't use right away, it stores in the body for later use as body fat. Despite our society's tradition of grand dinners, our bodies are much better equipped to process a larger meal in the morning or at lunch than in the evening. If you do not normally eat breakfast, eating a large meal first thing in the morning can seem logistically daunting or even physically sickening. Incorporate breakfast slowly by eating lighter and earlier dinners and small breakfasts, such as toast with nut butters, before transitioning to fuller, more nourishing morning meals. Your body will operate much more efficiently when you eat consistent meals and snacks regularly through the day instead of constantly underfueling and overfueling.

Many people reason that by skipping breakfast or skipping snacks, they'll eat fewer calories overall. The truth is that skipping meals and snacks actually makes you eat *more* by the end of the day. When you eventually sit down to a meal, you're so famished that you eat without listening to hunger or satiety cues. It seems counterintuitive, but eating smaller meals, more often is much healthier.

Ideally, provide your body with nourishment at least three times— breakfast, lunch, and dinner. You may find that if you are active, you get hungry in between meals or after workouts; snacking provides you with the fuel you need to stay awake and alert. Snacks are also an ideal time to squeeze in a serving of fruit or vegetables. For unique healthy snack ideas, check out pages 236–38.

But What About Calories?

It's logical that whole, unprocessed foods greatly contribute to your overall well-being. The more you process something, the less nutritious it becomes. It's obvious that eating correct serving sizes is important, too. And it makes sense that diets rooted in plants—whole grains, vegetables, and fruits—are more nutritious than diets filled with meat and sweets. But many people choose to focus on just one thing—calories.

I used to be a calorie cruncher, and I would make decisions about whether a food is healthy based solely on the food's calorie content. Calorie crunchers flip a box over and scan the first few lines of the nutrition facts label, using one number to decide if the food is "worth it." Entire Web sites are dedicated to helping people track their calories, while others rely on the old pen-and-paper method of counting. There are even smartphone apps that can calculate the caloric content of your meal by analyzing a picture of it!

Counting appeals to many people, but is it necessary—or even healthy? The answer to the calorie-countin' conundrum is complicated, so let's start from the beginning. . . .

Calories are simply a way to measure how much energy is in food. Some foods are more calorie dense than others because of their macronutrient content; protein and carbohydrates contain four calories per gram, while fats provide nine calories per gram. It makes sense that a dense piece of steak would have more calories than a juicy apple, since the steak has more protein and fat than the apple has carbohydrates, gram for gram.

Before we go any further, there's a dieting red flag that we need to talk about right now, before digging into calories and weight. Many diets preach that the trick to losing weight is shunning a particular macronutrient, like carbs or fats, but, more often than not, this technique is successful only because the dieter effectively slashes calories by avoiding the macronutrient in question. Avoidance of any macronutrient (or food group) is dangerous because it creates imbalance in your body. Protein, carbohydrates, and fats are *all* necessary for your basic biological functions. Protein is part of every cell—and therefore all the tissue, organs, and bones—in your body. Without protein, your body cannot repair itself. In addition to being a key part of the cell-building process, healthy fats aid in the absorption of some vitamins and nutrients. And last, carbohydrates provide your body with a readily available source of fuel. Moral of the story? Don't be afraid to eat any macronutrient!

If you don't immediately use up the calories you ingest, your body will store the extra energy . . . on your thighs, stomach, or backside: 3,500 unused calories are equal to one pound of stored body fat. As a sort of ancient biological insurance policy, calories that are not burned off by your body's metabolic processes hang around. Unfortunately, the human body simply hasn't gotten the memo that most Americans aren't exactly going days in between hunting-and-gathering expeditions.

That's why the general relationship between the calories in the foods you consume, the calories your body burns to stay alive, and any extra calories you burn through activity and exercise is so important. The amount of calories you eat and drink has a direct impact on your weight, regardless of whether those calories are healthy calories or not. If you overeat healthy food, you will still gain weight. If you undereat junk food, you might lose weight—you just won't be very healthy. Calories are also important to consider if you exercise regularly, because you'll need a general idea of how many calories you need to consume (and when) to power through your workout and aid in muscle recovery.

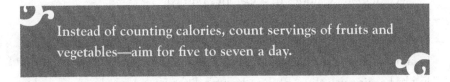

Instead of counting calories, count servings of fruits and vegetables—aim for five to seven a day.

Does this mean that calorie counting is essential to a Healthy Tipping Point? Of course not! Calorie counting is not ideal for everyone. I used calorie counting during the first six months of my healthy journey, but it quickly became annoying and tedious—a common compliant. Additionally, if you've suffered from distorted eating or thinking in the past, fixating on calories can be dangerous. Many people find counting brings out their worst perfectionist behaviors and stirs up all those distorted feelings in a new way. Third, counting calories can take the focus off of where it belongs—eating a balanced diet of mainly whole, unprocessed foods and relying on your body's hunger cues to drive your eating habits. Counters might begin to believe a 100-calorie cookie is nutritionally equivalent to a 100-calorie apple. And last, calorie counting can teach you to ignore your hunger—or satiety—cues. After all, what if you've reached your calorie limit for the day but are still hungry? Or what if you're 100 calories under your limit but feel totally stuffed—do you force yourself to eat more?

Clearly, the relationship between calories and physical and mental health is complex. You may choose to count temporarily to gain a better understanding of your intake needs, count for the long term to help you stay on track, or choose not to count at all and focus on simply eating a balanced, plant-based diet of real food. Regardless, a basic understanding of calories—and by extension, portion sizes—is a powerful tool for long-term health.

The mathematical equations for the relationship between weight loss, gain, or maintenance and calories are quite simple (on paper, that is—in real life, it can be much more complex!):

Weight Maintenance: Calories In = Calories Burned
Weight Loss: Calories In < Calories Burned
Weight Gain: Calories In > Calories Burned

To apply one of these formulas to your life, you must first calculate your basal metabolic rate (BMR), which is how many calories your body burns just by keeping you alive. BMRs adjust for differences due to height, weight, age, and gender. The formula for BMR follows:

Non-pregnant women: BMR = 655 + (4.35 × weight in pounds) +
(4.7 × height in inches)–(4.7 × age in years)

Men: BMR = 66 + (6.23 × weight in pounds) + (12.7 × height in
inches)−(6.8 × age in years)

Based on this formula, a thirty-year-old woman who is five foot five
inches and 150 pounds needs to consume 1,472 calories a day *just* to maintain basic body functions. Regularly dipping below your BMR is, obviously,
extremely dangerous to your health.

Your caloric needs are greater than your BMR because most of us don't
lie in bed all day long—we move! To determine your total average daily
calorie needs, multiply your BMR by the appropriate activity factor (known
as the Harris Benedict equation):

Sedentary (little or no exercise; office job): BMR × 1.2
Lightly active (light exercise/sports one to three days/week):
     BMR × 1.375
Moderately active (moderate exercise/sports three to five days/week):
     BMR × 1.55
Very active (hard exercise/sports six to seven days a week):
     BMR × 1.725
Extra active (hard exercise/sports multiple times a day or a physically
     demanding job): BMR × 1.9

If our friend in the example above worked in an office and never exercised, she would need to eat 1,766 calories a day to maintain her weight. If
she read this book and got motivated to run a 5K and trained three days a
week, she would need to eat somewhere between 2,024 calories (BMR ×
1.375) and 2,281 calories (BMR × 1.55) *every day*—not just on days she
worked out—to maintain her weight. And, if after running her 5K, our gal
added two days of swimming and strength training to her weekly workouts,
she would need to increase her daily calories even more to maintain her
weight.

This example raises an important point: if you're not looking to lose
weight and begin an exercise program or step up your workouts, you'll need

to add calories to your diet to make sure you're fueled properly. Otherwise, you increase your risk for short- and long-term health problems, including workout-related injuries. One reason for this increased risk of injury is that, if you aren't eating enough calories, your body won't have the energy to repair stressed muscles. If you are very active and find that you're hungry on hard exercise days, you may find that it's necessary to eat a few hundred additional calories on top of the recommended amount—honor your body's needs! Choose a snack that is rich in protein and fat, not just straight carbohydrates, because this will help satiate your hunger—a slice of peanut butter toast should do the trick. Food is fuel! Remember that these calculations are just guidelines, not gospel.

On the flip side, if you are looking to lose weight, you'll want to create a small calorie deficit each day. A bigger goal is not better in this scenario, either. Losing weight too quickly is dangerous, and even if you have a lot of weight to lose, chronic underfueling is unhealthy. Slow and steady is not only safer, it's more maintainable (because who wants to go through life without dessert?!). Most experts agree that a weight loss of one to two pounds a week is a healthy rate; if you're obese, your doctor can tell you if it's okay to lose weight faster during the first few weeks of your lifestyle transformation.

Since a pound of body fat equals 3,500 calories, a person can lose one pound in seven days through creating a calorie deficit of 500 calories a day. You can do this through exercise (calorie counts of common exercises can be found online or you can use a heart-rate monitor to estimate your calories burned). It's important to remember that exercise alone is not usually an effective weight-loss tool. When people increase their physical activity, they tend to experience an increase in appetite. For most people, losing weight requires nutritional changes as well.

As an example, let's say our previously mentioned friend, who works in an office and doesn't exercise, wanted to lose weight. If she continued to eat 1,766 calories a day and didn't exercise, she would maintain her weight. If she ate 250 fewer calories (1,516) and burned 250 calories a day through exercise, she would lose a pound a week. If she chose not to exercise, it would be unwise to unload 500 calories from her diet each day; she would drop below her BMR and probably gnaw off her arm out of hunger. A safer route would be to simply lose weight at a slower, safer speed.

It's important to note that calorie calculations, calories burned during exercise, and even calorie counts on nutritional labels are just estimates (a nutritional label may say there is eight ounces in the package, but there might be seven or nine, for example!). These equations and numbers are only provided as a place to start; you'll have to adjust your diet and exercise in response to your results. Having a basic understanding about how calories impact your weight and health is an invaluable tool, but at the end of the day, healthy eating is about so much more.

And just as healthy eating is about more than calories, healthy living— and experiencing your Healthy Tipping Point—is about way more than the foods you eat. It's about finding emotional peace and self-confidence. For some, this might mean *never, ever calorie counting*. Healthy living is also about exercising, not just for weight management, but for general wellness, too. Many Healthy Tipping Points occur when a person realizes that health is really about what's on the inside. They eat better and exercise more than before, but perhaps the scale doesn't flash back their goal number, and they're okay with that. Remember this: your weight isn't a surefire indicator of your holistic health. You are more than a number on the scale or the sum of your caloric intake.

Six

HEALTHY EATING SPECIFICS

Nutrients for a Healthier Body

While it's great to know the biological reasons behind why you should make certain food choices, all of that information can seem overwhelming, too. So before we get into the nitty-gritty on some key nutrients for a healthier body, maybe it's best to sum up the Healthy Tipping Point style of eating with a visual—a plate.

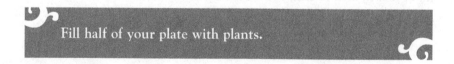

Fill half of your plate with plants.

On a plant-based diet, the focus is nutrient-rich plants—vegetables, fruits, and grains, as well as nuts, seeds, and oils in lesser amounts. These plants should fill up the majority of your plate. Animal protein and dairy may have a place on your plate, but they're not the star of the show. When I plate my meals, I try to imagine my dinner plate like a pie chart and give plants *at least* half of the pie. Varying the types of vegetables and fruits, grains, nuts, seeds, animal protein, dairy, and oils that you eat each day will also ensure you're getting enough of the basic nutrients your body needs to thrive. This simple little visualization will help you serve up proper portions, eat more plants, and reduce your meat and sweets consumption.

PROTEIN, CALCIUM, OMEGA-3S—OH MY!

This section includes a lot of scientific information on healthy eating. You might find this interesting and illuminating or totally overwhelming, especially if this style of eating is a major shift from what you're used to. If you feel swamped with stats, just remember that it all boils down to three things: eating more plants, eating a variety of real foods, and eating correct portion sizes. That's it! If you do these three simple things, you're eating a healthier diet.

This section provides a deeper look into how key nutrients influence your health. We'll also bust some common myths about these nutrients.

Healthy Tipping Point Success Story: Amy, 37, Utah

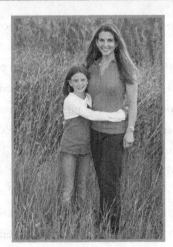

Just after graduating college, I got a job at the state department of health. I counseled state employees on healthy habits, including eating well, which I could relate to because I was on my journey to lose thirty pounds. Many of my clients had children, and they would pick up fast food for dinner and send processed foods for lunch and snacks to day care. They wanted to feed their kids better, but didn't feel like they had the time or energy.

One year later, I had my first child. I

was determined to feed him the way I encouraged my clients to feed their children. I found out it was *much* harder than I thought it would be. Years passed, and my family grew. In the middle of a meal with my kids, I was struggling to explain why they should eat fruits and vegetables. Then, I had an idea. I grabbed a divided plate from the pantry and pointed to the largest section—half your meal should be fruits and veggies, I explained. I told my kids that if half the plate is full of plants, you feel happier. I created a plate with a picture in each section to drive home the concept. They were thrilled. Instead of complaining, they actually asked to fill up their plates with more fruits and vegetables!

I created the Healthy Habits Kids Food Plate (www.healthykidsplate .com), an easy tool that teaches children about properly balanced and healthy meals. The plate is divided into three sections that each feature a fun cartoon design of healthy foods: fruits and veggies; proteins like eggs or chicken; and carbohydrates like pasta, bread, and pretzels. I really think kids will eventually develop a taste for healthy foods, if you continue to serve them.

PROTEIN

We live in a meat-focused society, so it's no surprise that the most common question posed to plant-based eaters is, "But where do you get your protein?!" In fact, this might be one of *your* primary concerns as you switch to a greener diet. After all, protein is *essential* to human life. Your body needs protein to grow, repair, and regenerate. Your muscles are comprised primarily of protein, and the macronutrient is also a major player in the health of your teeth, hormones, enzymes, organs, bones, skin, hair, and blood.

Americans have a cultural bias toward animal-protein sources that is reinforced by the food industry and the government for a variety of complex political and economic reasons. Diet gurus tout high-protein diets as a miraculous weight-loss tool. Health stores push protein shakes and protein bars. Restaurants dedicate sections of their menu to high-protein specials. There's a lot of hype about protein, so it's not surprising that people tend to focus on "the protein question" when switching to a plant-based diet.

However, the concern about plant-based eaters being protein deficient is mostly unfounded. In fact, the United States Department of Agriculture (USDA) states that "inadequate protein intake in the United States is rare."[11] Most Americans actually eat too much protein, which can cause kidney issues. Protein is in almost everything we eat—including fruits, vegetables, and whole grains (yes, there's even protein in bread!). And although protein is important, a greater proportion of your calories should come from carbohydrates and fat. As a reminder, a gram of protein and a gram of carbohydrates equal four calories, but a gram of fat equals nine calories. This means you'll eat fewer grams of fat than grams of protein, but a higher proportion of your calories will come from fat.

Diets like Atkins or South Beach have convinced many people that the key to weight loss is a high-protein plan; however, there is strong evidence that caloric intake matters more than the proportion of macronutrients. In fact, research by the USDA has found that eating a high-protein/low-carb diet is statistically no more effective for weight loss than a diet that is, say, 65 percent carbohydrates, 15 percent protein, and 20 percent fat.[12] There is no magically perfect proportion of carbs/proteins/fats when it comes to weight loss or weight maintenance. It's really all about your caloric intake.

A general rule of thumb for daily protein intake is that people who are maintaining their weight should eat at least 0.8 gram of protein for every kilogram of body weight.

Your weight in pounds / 2.2 = Your weight in kilograms
Your weight in kilograms × 0.8 grams of protein = Your minimum daily
    protein requirement

Thus, a 120-pound person needs at least forty-three grams of protein, a 150-pound person needs fifty-five grams of protein, and a 200-pound person needs seventy-two grams of protein. Although a diet higher in protein isn't necessary for weight loss, some people find that they feel fuller when they eat a higher percentage of their calories from protein. To help increase feelings of satiety on a diet, some dietitians suggest aiming for up to 25 percent of calories from protein.

PROTEIN AND ATHLETES

Muscle needs protein to repair and grow, which is why people who are active often believe they need more protein. Remember that the more active you are, the more calories you need to consume; thus, you'll naturally eat more protein. As an example, a 150-pound marathoner may eat around 2,800 calories a day. If 10 percent of these calories came from protein (the same proportion as before), she'd eat seventy grams of protein. This works out to approximately 1.0 grams of protein per kilogram of body weight.

If you're extremely active, many nutrition experts will recommend you strive for a slightly higher percentage of protein in your diet, such as 1.0–1.2 grams of protein per kilogram of body weight to assist with muscle recovery.

For people who are lightly or moderately active, it's not necessary to up your percentage of protein, but it is important to time your intake of protein for maximum muscle recovery. Check out page 257 for more information.

Whew! All of this math might be making your head swim. If so, don't worry. The bottom line is that it's actually very easy to meet your minimum needs (0.8 grams per kilogram of body weight or 10 percent of your total calories) just by eating a varied, plant-based diet.

This warrants repeating: if you're eating enough calories and eating lots of different foods, counting protein grams is usually completely unnecessary.

Remember—a plant-based diet doesn't mean you have to give up meat, poultry, or fish entirely if you don't want to; it's about simply *eating more plants.* A plant-based diet can deliver the protein that you need to stay healthy and strong. It is entirely possible—and desirable for long-term health—to get a majority of your protein needs from plant-protein sources because these foods are generally lower in saturated fat and cholesterol free. Plus, plant-protein sources offer other important nutrients—like vitamins and minerals—bite by bite!

PLANT-BASED PROTEIN SOURCES

Food	Approximate Grams of Protein
¼ cup hummus	2.0
3 ounces wild salmon	18.0
½ cup chickpeas	6.0
½ cup black beans	7.0
½ avocado	1.75
1 cup cooked quinoa	6.0
1 cup cooked brown rice	4.5
1 cup kale, measured raw	2.5
1 veggie burger	5.0–15.0
1 egg	6.5
4 ounces organic grass-fed beef	23.0
1 slice whole wheat bread	3.0–5.0
⅓ (15-ounce) package extra-firm tofu	13.2
1 ounce nuts	3.0–7.0
1 sweet potato	4.0
1 cup legumes	5.0–9.0
2 tablespoons nut butter (peanut, cashew, almond, sunflower)	3.0–8.0
1 cup soy milk	7.0
1 cup almond milk	1.0
1 cup 2 percent cow's milk	8.0
1 banana	1.3
½ cup dry old-fashioned oats	5.0

Food	Approximate Grams of Protein
4 ounces organic turkey breast	23.0
6 ounces plain, nonfat Greek yogurt	15.0–18.0
1 (6-ounce) container organic low-fat vanilla yogurt	7.0
1 ounce cheddar cheese	7.0
2 tablespoons ground flaxseed	3.0

Source: CalorieCount.com

Now that we've established that getting enough protein on a plant-based diet isn't a problem, let's break down some other common protein myths:

MYTH

- **Plant-based diets lack the key amino acids that animal protein provides:** Dietary protein is a combination of amino acids. Scientists have identified nine essential amino acids that a healthy diet must include because our bodies cannot produce them.

  When people say that animal protein is a "complete" protein, they really mean that animal protein (dairy and meat) naturally contains all nine essential amino acids. Some plant protein sources contain all of the essential amino acids, but the amount of one or two amino acids might be low. Other plant protein sources are completely missing several essential amino acids. However, there are no amino acids that are present only in animal protein sources, so it's entirely possible to eat a very strict plant-based diet, such as veganism, and get all the amino acids your body needs.

MYTH

- **Plant-based diets must combine certain foods to get complete proteins:** This myth is based on the truth that most plant protein sources are lacking at least one essential amino acid. Many people believe that you must combine certain foods at meals to get a complete protein if you choose not to eat animal protein sources. The theory of complementary protein is a lot like a jigsaw puzzle—if you eat le-gumes, which are low in the essential amino acid methionine, you should eat a food that is high in methionine, such as whole wheat, at the same meal. When put together, the legumes and the whole wheat provide your body with all nine essential amino acids.

In the 1970s, the USDA preached that food combining was abso-lutely necessary to achieve a healthy plant-based diet, but the practice has been largely debunked. Your body temporarily stores the amino acids you ingest and draws on them when needed. Thus, the most important thing is to eat a *variety* of healthy foods every day.

AWESOME NUTS AND SEEDS

Nuts and seeds are especially important for plant-based eaters. Not only is this dynamic duo a healthy source of protein and fat, but some—like pump-kin seeds, pistachios, cashews, and hemp seeds—even provide the body with all nine essential amino acids in the proper ratios, just like meat or dairy.[13] Nuts and seeds are typically nutrient- *and* calorie-dense; a handful a day is usually the perfect amount.

MYTH

- **Protein powders are a perfect real-food protein substitute:** There are several different types of protein supplements, some of which are animal based and others that are plant based. The most common type of protein powder is whey, which is derived from dairy. There are also soy, egg, hemp seed, pea, and rice protein powders. You can buy many of these plant-based protein powders online or in specialty grocery stores such as Whole Foods.

  Protein powder is, by definition, a fake and processed food; how-ever, some brands are more real than others. Many brands contain artificial coloring, preservatives, and artificial sweeteners, including acesulfame potassium, aspartame, neotame, saccharin, and sucralose. Additionally, most brands include conventionally grown, nonorganic ingredients and can contain trace amounts of pesticides, antibiotics, and other chemicals.

Protein powder is definitely not the ideal real-food protein substitute; however, in the real world, protein powders are simply more convenient than other protein sources—following a hard workout, it's easier and faster to whip up a smoothie with some rice protein powder than it is to grill up a fillet of salmon. If protein powders fit into your lifestyle, make sure you read ingredient labels and select the protein powder with the most real-food ingredients; choose organic protein powders when possible; and consume protein powder in moderation. Additionally, by switching the type of protein powder you purchase— for example, buying brown rice protein powder when your whey runs out, and then opting for hemp seed powder—you'll ingest a greater variety of nutrients over the long term.

MYTH

- **Soy is a perfect meat substitute:** When seeking out a plant alternative to animal protein, many people naturally reach for soy products, including tofu, TVP (textured vegetable protein—the stuff faux chicken and faux beef is made from), tempeh, soy yogurt and ice cream, soy cheese, and soy milk. You might have even eaten whole soybeans at Japanese restaurants before—the appetizer is called edamame.

Soy seems to be a double-edged sword. There are many benefits to eating soy—it's high in protein, is thought to contain all the essential amino acids, and is a source of alpha-linolenic acid omega-3s (for more on omega-3s, see page 145). On the other hand, many critics say that soy can introduce danger into a diet. Soy is one naturally occurring source of phytoestrogens, which can negatively influence the delicate balance of estrogens in the body if ingested in extremely high amounts. Women who are at a high risk of developing certain cancers, especially breast cancer, are frequently warned to avoid soy. However, some large-scale studies have indicated that phytoestrogens can have a preventive effect on breast, endometrial, and prostate cancer; decrease the risk of cardiovascular disease; and prevent osteoporosis.

Thus, whether soy is unhealthy really depends on the amount and your risk factors for certain cancers, especially breast cancer.[14] It is generally considered safe for people with an average risk of breast cancer to eat moderate amounts of soy products—just remember that soy is added to a lot of foods that you wouldn't expect to find it in, such as granola bars and cereals. Limiting yourself to eating soy products three times a week is probably prudent. Plus, many soy products are highly processed, which is another reason to eat soy only in moderation.

For a detailed explanation on how to buy and prepare tofu, see page 189.

SOY-FREE MEAT ALTERNATIVES

Instead of tofu or faux soy meat, try these soy-free meat alternatives in your favorite recaps:

- **Seitan:** Pronounced say-tahn, seitan is made from wheat, but it tastes more like meat than bread! Seitan is made by rinsing wheat flour dough with water until all the starch dissolves. Seitan is high in protein (about eighteen grams per serving). Seitan is denser than tofu and is often used in faux chicken or beef recipes at Chinese restaurants. You can find seitan products near the tofu in your grocer's refrigerated section.
- **Beans:** Above all else, beans are cheap! Kidney beans, navy beans, black beans, chickpeas, and other types of beans are a great real-food alternative to meat in soups, chili, burritos, salads, rice bowls, and even sandwiches. If you buy canned beans to save preparation time, make sure you drain and rinse the beans first—one study found that the process removes an average of 41 percent of the sodium.[15]
- **Lentils:** With eighteen grams of protein per cooked cup, lentils are another inexpensive source of plant protein. Actually a seed, lentils come

in many different colors (red, green, and brown) and taste wonderful with rice and a flavorful curry sauce.

Another great option is tempeh, which is created from soybeans but is less processed than tofu. Tempeh is higher in protein and fiber than tofu and tastes slightly nutty or earthy.

Healthy Tipping Point Success Story: Matt, 30, Maryland

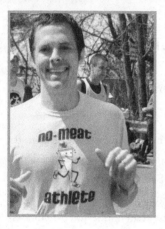

With four miles left in the marathon I had trained so hard for, I didn't think I'd make it. It wasn't finishing I was worried about—I was trying to finish fast enough to qualify for the Boston Marathon. I had run many other marathons, but never fast enough to win a slot in the nation's most prestigious marathon. Just six months prior, I had completely changed my diet. It was a big risk, considering it's almost a given among athletes that eating lots of lean meat for protein is the way to build strength and speed. At first, my reasons for going vegetarian were more about compassion than fitness: I just didn't feel right about eating animals anymore. But barely a few weeks into my new diet, I realized there was much more to it than that. I noticed I was running and recovering faster than I ever had before.

But I wasn't sure if it was enough—after all, to qualify for the Boston Marathon, I would have to finish under three hours and eleven minutes—a 7:17-minute-per-mile pace for 26.2 miles. It was something I had tried unsuccessfully to do for seven years, and here I was, with four miles to go . . .

only this time, that sharp decline held off. Somewhere, I found the strength to push harder, actually speeding up during those final few miles. As I turned into the wind one final time before the homestretch, I knew I had done it. I finished the race in 3:09:59, and I'm not a bit ashamed to admit that when I hugged my wife at the finish, my eyes welled up with tears as I told her, "I did it."

Was it the vegetarian diet that did it for me? Maybe, but it wasn't just that. It was the work, not just that summer, but in the seven years since I had run my first marathon, almost two hours slower. But without a doubt, I know that the plant-based diet is what gave me the energy to work so hard in the months leading up to the race—for my body, this diet worked. Two years later, I'm still vegetarian (actually vegan now), and I've never felt better. Sure, I don't get 150 grams of protein a day like I used to when I ate chicken breasts and steaks, but I now understand what a ridiculous amount of protein that is! Best of all, this diet has forced me to eat the one thing that somehow never made it onto my plate before—fresh vegetables.

And every time I realize, out of the blue and as if it's news, that I don't eat animals anymore, I remember the reason I did this in the first place: for the animals. And that, more than the fitness or even the long-term health benefits, is why I continue to eat this way.

IRON

Iron is an important mineral in any healthy diet because iron carries oxygen in your blood to every cell in your body. Iron also supports a healthy immune system. There are two types of iron: heme iron and nonheme iron. Heme iron comes from meat, poultry, and fish; nonheme iron comes from plants. An excess of either type of iron is dangerous because of the mineral's propensity to oxidize and produce free radicals, which can cause a host of health issues like cardiovascular disease, cancer, and other inflammatory conditions. It's actually easier to overdo it on heme iron because that type is more readily absorbed by your body. In fact, if you're eating a variety of iron-rich foods, it's probably unnecessary (or even potentially harmful) to take an iron supplement if you don't have an identified iron deficiency or medical condition that necessitates the intake of extra iron.

To ensure you get the right amount of iron in your diet, you'll want to do three things: eat a variety of iron-rich foods, eat iron-rich food with iron enhancers, and minimize iron inhibitors when eating iron-rich foods.

- **Eat a Variety of Iron-Rich Foods:** Each day, men and nonmenstruating women require about ten to fourteen milligrams, menstruating or nursing women need fifteen to thirty milligrams, and pregnant women need about thirty milligrams of iron. However, counting milligrams of iron is unrealistic, so just focus on eating iron-rich foods every day.

  When most people hear "iron," they think, "beef!" Other foods rich in iron include dark leafy green vegetables (spinach, chard, turnip greens, collard greens, mustard greens), as well as blackstrap molasses, romaine lettuce, string beans, Brussels sprouts, asparagus, chickpeas, broccoli, leeks, kelp, lentils, whole grains, nuts and seeds, lima beans, pinto beans, navy beans, sweet potato, tofu, and many, many other tasty real foods. Spices such as thyme, dill weed, parsley, basil, cinnamon, rosemary, oregano, and turmeric provide 1 milligram to 3.5 milligrams of iron per two-tablespoon serving.

- **Eat Iron-Rich Foods with Iron Enhancers:** The bioavailability of nonheme iron in food (how easily your body absorbs a substance into your bloodstream) is greatly influenced by the other foods you eat in the same meal. Absorption of nonheme iron is enhanced when eaten with foods that are rich in vitamin C, including oranges; lemons; kiwis; grapefruit; tomatoes; broccoli; and red, orange, or green peppers. This sounds more complicated in theory than it does in practice—you probably do this already without even realizing it! A summer salad with spinach, mandarin oranges, strawberries, and black beans is a perfect mix of iron-rich foods and iron enhancers.

> To promote healthy digestion, drink a glass of water before eating breakfast, and wait to drink tea or coffee until after—not during—the meal.

- **Minimize Iron Inhibitors When Eating Iron-Rich Foods:** Just as some foods increase the bioavailability of iron, other foods minimize it. The tannic acid in tea is one common culprit. Coffee has a similar inhibiting effect. If you do drink tea or coffee, drink it in between meals to minimize its inhibiting effect. Calcium also inhibits the absorption of iron; if you take a calcium supplement, take it in between meals.

SYMPTOMS OF ANEMIA

Anemia is a medical condition when your blood lacks enough red blood cells and hemoglobin; as a result, your muscles and organs don't get enough oxygen. People associate anemia with not getting enough iron, but anemia can also occur if an individual is deficient in vitamin B_{12}; has experienced chronic lead poisoning; or has a medical condition such as ulcers, jaundice, gallstones, sickle cell anemia, and more. General warning signs for anemia include feeling tired or weak, a rapid heart rate, dizziness, cramping in the legs, insomnia, and difficulty concentrating. If you suspect you have anemia, your doctor can confirm the type of anemia and the cause through blood tests.

CALCIUM AND VITAMIN D

It's not exactly news that adequate calcium in your diet is extremely important. But most Americans have been brainwashed by the dairy industry to believe the only way to get enough calcium is to drink several glasses of milk each day. In reality, milk isn't the only or even the best—considering regular dairy's high saturated fat content—natural source of calcium. Beyond low or nonfat dairy, other healthy sources of calcium include dark leafy greens (such as collard greens, Swiss chard, kale); broccoli; most brands of tofu; green beans; green peas; sesame seeds; blackstrap molasses; and almonds.

FOR THE LADIES

One research study of more than 440 women suffering from PMS found that taking 1,200 milligrams of calcium carbonate daily reduced by 48 percent the severity of premenstrual symptoms, such as mood swings and cramping, by the third cycle.[16] Calcium can negatively interact with certain medications, so be sure to get a doctor's okay before taking a supplement.

Calcium intake is important for several reasons, but especially because it helps prevent bone loss and osteoporosis, which is *not* just a concern for the elderly. Bone density peaks in your early thirties; without enough dietary calcium, your body will harvest the calcium from your bones to support basic biological functions, like muscle and nerve function.

The recommended daily allowance for calcium:

- Teens: 1,300 milligrams
- Adults (19–50 years old): 1,000 milligrams
- Older adults (over 50 years old): 1,000 milligrams for men and 1,300 milligrams for women

If you're eating a variety of foods, including lots of plants, it's pretty easy to get enough calcium through your diet alone. For example, a meal of one cup of steamed collard greens, three ounces of firm tofu, a handful of chopped almonds, and brown rice topped with salsa contains about 500 milligrams of calcium—half your daily need.

DAIRY ALTERNATIVES

Whether you're lactose intolerant or just want to reduce your animal product consumption, there are many healthy, real-food alternatives to meat and traditional dairy products like yogurt and cheese.

The amount of naturally occurring calcium in many of these dairy alternatives is low; however, manufacturers usually fortify their products with added calcium and vitamin D—just check the nutritional label (for reference, one cup of skim milk has 300 milligrams of calcium). You'll always want to thoroughly read the ingredients list to check for an excess of fake-food ingredients. Just because an item is dairy free doesn't automatically mean it's healthy!

- **Milk:** Nondairy milk alternatives include soy milk, rice milk, almond milk, hemp milk, and oat milk. Popular brands are Silk, Almond Breeze, and Rice Dream, and many milk alternatives can be found in the refrigerated section or on the shelf in the organic section of your regular grocery store. Generally, soy and almond milk tend to be the creamiest and best for cereals; rice, hemp, and oat milk may be thinner and tastiest in baked goods or smoothies.
- **Cheese:** Nondairy shredded and sliced cheese and cream cheese alternatives are often crafted from soy/tofu, cashews, potato starch, or tapioca. National brands include Daiya, Follow Your Heart, and Vegan Gourmet. A great real-food alternative to faux cheese is hummus, which you can mix into casseroles or spread on sandwiches.
- **Butter:** Most manufacturers of margarine have removed trans fat from their ingredient lists; however, most brands still contain dairy. Nondairy alternatives are crafted from soy or oil blends (such as olive, coconut, or canola oil). Earth Balance is one popular brand.

> • **Yogurt:** Beyond cow- and goat-milk yogurt (people who are slightly al-
> lergic to lactose can often tolerate goat milk), there is soy yogurt and
> coconut milk yogurt. Popular brands include So Delicious, Silk, and
> WholeSoy.

And just like iron, calcium has a few enhancers and inhibitors. Eating excessive protein and salt may trigger calcium excretion in the kidneys—yet
another reason to eat a moderate, plant-based diet. On the other hand,
vitamin D helps your body process the calcium that you eat. Without adequate vitamin D, your body will harvest the calcium it needs from your
bones, even if you're eating calcium-rich foods. Inadequate vitamin D intake can also contribute to heart disease, decreased immune function, and
other chronic health issues.[17]

Vitamin D is nicknamed the sunshine vitamin because the primary
way our body receives it is by simply being outside. When in contact with
the skin, ultraviolet B rays initiate a process that converts cholesterol in the
skin to vitamin D_3. It's estimated that one billion people are vitamin-D
deficient, and part of the problem is that people spend more time indoors
than ever before, and when they do go outside, they slather on sunscreen
immediately. Due to fears about skin cancer, we've been convinced that
sunshine is always bad—but it's not. In fact, it's absolutely necessary!

For most Americans (except those in the southernmost states), it can
be difficult or impossible to get vitamin D through sunshine all year long,
since the sun never gets high enough in the sky for its ultraviolet B rays to
penetrate the atmosphere during the winter. But in the summer, it's easy to
soak up vitamin D. A light-skinned person with their arms and legs exposed
will trigger the manufacture of approximately 10,000 international units
(IUs) of vitamin D in a few minutes, many times the government's minimum recommended amount. See what I did there? Yup—I just gave you an
excuse to step outside and enjoy the sunshine. Soak it up!

In the middle of summer, fair-skinned people should be outside for only a few minutes before covering up or putting on sunscreen, but dark-skinned people or elderly persons naturally produce less vitamin D in response to sunshine and may need to be outside longer to get the same positive effect.[18] While your body can store up vitamin D from the summer, people who live in the north will run out of their banked amounts by late winter. Depending on where you live and your skin tone, it may be necessary to take a vitamin D supplement. Your doctor can run a blood test to check for vitamin D deficiency.

THE RIGHT VITAMIN D SUPPLEMENT

When taking a vitamin D supplement, choose a supplement that contains vitamin D_3 (cholecalciferol) instead of vitamin D_2 (ergocalciferol). Cholecalciferol is three to four times more potent. You should first take a blood test to confirm a deficiency, and as always, check with your doctor before taking any supplements.

OMEGA-3 FATTY ACIDS

Omega-3 fatty acids are considered one of the essential fatty acids because your body cannot produce them, just like the nine essential amino acids. Omega-3s play an important role in brain function, mood stabilization, growth, and development; there is also significant research that omega-3s may reduce the risk of heart disease, decrease inflammation throughout the body, and lower the risk of other chronic diseases, such as asthma, cancer, and arthritis. The jury is still out on how the intake of another essential fatty acid—omega-6s—in relation to omega-3s impacts your health. However, one thing is clear: omega-3s are definitely part of a healthy diet.

There are actually two critical types of omega-3 fatty acids that your body needs: eicosapentaenoic acid (EPA) and docosahexaenoic (DHA). EPA and DHA are found almost exclusively in cold-water fish, including

salmon, sardines, herring, mackerel, black cod, and bluefish. A third type
of omega-3 fatty acid is called alpha-linolenic acid (ALA); ALA comes
exclusively from plants. If you choose not to eat fish or simply don't regularly eat mackerel—never fear. Your body is capable of converting a portion
of ALA to EPA and DHA!

SOURCES OF OMEGA-3S

EPA	DHA	ALA
Whole fish or fish oils from cod liver, her-ring, trout, mackerel, salmon, menhaden, sardine, bluefin tuna, crab, scallops, lob-ster, tilapia, and shrimp		Ground flaxseed, flaxseed oil, canola oil, soybeans, pine nuts, wheat germ, kidney beans, pinto beans, mung beans, chia seeds, hemp seeds, walnuts, pecans, hazel-nuts, broccoli, spinach, winter squashes

As omega-3s have become more and more recognized as a key component
of a healthy diet, fish oil supplements (or DHA/EPA vegan algae supplements; the fish get their omega-3s from algae) have become widely popular
in recent years. But before you reach for that supplement, know this: research suggests that omega-3s from whole-food sources are more readily
absorbed by the body than omega-3s from supplements.

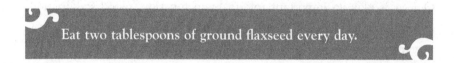

Eat two tablespoons of ground flaxseed every day.

Omega-3s sound complicated and overwhelming. But really, it's easy to
get omega-3s in your diet: just add two tablespoons of nutty-tasting ground
flaxseed (or chia seeds, another great source of plant-based omega-3s) to
your cereal, yogurt, smoothie, or oatmeal each day for a healthy dose of

ALA. Be sure to drink a glass of water at the same time, since hydration is important to ensure you digest these omega-3 essential fatty acids properly. Bonus points: two tablespoons of ground flaxseed contains four grams of fiber!

Because your body cannot digest whole flaxseeds, grind your own in small batches or seek out preground flaxseed in special mylar packaging, which helps the flax maintain its nutritional properties in a way that regular plastic cannot. Store preground flaxseed in the refrigerator to keep it from going rancid too quickly. (As always with any significant nutritional shift, check with your doctor before adding flaxseed to your diet. Ground flaxseed can interact negatively with some medications and medical conditions, including diabetes.)[19]

SUPPLEMENTS

Vitamins and supplements cannot replace a healthy, plant-based diet; however, supplements do serve an important purpose. Some people can struggle to get enough of certain nutrients despite their healthy diet. This can be due to the time of the year—as in the case of vitamin D—or because their bodies cannot effectively process all of the nutrients in the food they eat. Stress can have a significant impact on your body's ability to absorb nutrients. Pregnant women or people who are very active may also need supplementation, even on top of a healthy diet. Some people might even be lacking in key nutrients simply because the other foods they eat at the same time block absorption of the nutrient, like iron-rich foods and tea! And, of course, many people suffer from medical conditions that necessitate extra nutrients, not just the minimum recommended intake.

VEGANS AND VITAMIN B$_{12}$

Vitamin B$_{12}$ is an important nutrient found in animal products, including meat, fish, eggs, milk, and milk products. Some vegetarians and many vegans, who do not eat eggs, may struggle to make sure they receive adequate amounts of vitamin B$_{12}$. Fortunately, most breakfast cereals are fortified with vitamin B$_{12}$. Another source is fortified brewer's and nutritional yeasts, which can be sprinkled on veggies or used in sauces. Keep in mind that vitamin B$_{12}$ is light sensitive. Skip the brewer's and nutritional yeasts from the clear bulk bins at the health food stores, and store opaque containers of fortified brewer's and nutritional yeasts in the fridge or freezer to maximize its nutritional potential.

Alternatively, vegetarians and vegans may want to take a vitamin B$_{12}$ supplement.

All vitamins and supplements are not created equal. Like beauty products, the government exercises very little regulatory control over supplements. In fact, the government doesn't even consider supplements as medicine; in the FDA's eyes, supplements are a food product and thus subject to more relaxed regulation. And just like food, vitamins and supplements come in "real" and "fake" versions. Most of the supplements you see in stores (and the vitamins and minerals used to fortify foods) are created in pharmaceutical supplement labs. The vitamins and supplements are made from isolated fragments of nutrients; this is how manufacturers pack in 1,000 percent of your daily need in one small pill. These supplements are essentially Frankenvitamins! While this doesn't necessarily mean they are harmful to your health, it does mean these vitamins are not natural substances and thus not as easily assimilated by your body.

A NATURAL NAUSEA CURE

Ginger has been used for thousands of years as a natural cure for an upset stomach, headaches, and nausea. In fact, ginger is widely recognized as an excellent cure for pregnancy-related morning sickness and motion sickness. To make a ginger tea, peel and coarsely chop one inch of gingerroot, and then let it steep in a teapot of hot water for at least twenty minutes before drinking a cup or two. The tea also tastes wonderful with crushed fresh basil leaves.

The more natural, healthy alternative is whole-food supplements. These supplements are created from real foods; this means that you'll be able to recognize most of the ingredients on the label. Whole-food supplements are derived from plants, like carrots, beets, and kale, as well as animal products, like liver or blood proteins. Because these supplements are made from real ingredients, they can't be packed as tightly as isolated fragments. That means you may have to take more pills to reach your daily needs.

Whole-food supplements have limited availability; however, they are sold online and at traditional and alternative doctors' offices. In fact, many licensed holistic health-care providers—including naturopathic doctors, acupuncturists, and some chiropractors—specialize in providing supplement consultation and recommendations, so if you're not sure what kind of supplements you should be taking, consider working with traditional and alternative providers to get the most integrative care possible.

Greener Living

And by "green," I'm not talking about broccoli and spinach!

The green industry—organic, local, and natural produce and products—has exploded during the last two decades, climbing from one billion dollars

in sales in 1990 to $26.7 billion in 2010. More than 4.8 million acres of
American soil is devoted to organic farming, and while fresh produce is the
top-selling organic sector, 2.7 percent of dairy cows and 1.5 percent of egg-
laying hens are managed under the organic system. In 2008, green cleaning
products accounted for 3 percent of total market share—but will likely rise
to 30 percent by 2013.[20] The numbers speak for themselves—clearly, green
is a very big business.

As the industry booms, potential for abuse of customers' trust rises.
While the organic label is regulated by the USDA, other terms—natural,
pure, farm-fresh, free roam—are much more ambivalent and are used to
play to customer concerns about food sources, animal treatment, and purity
of ingredients.

READING BETWEEN THE LINES

When you're trying to make better food choices, it's difficult to distinguish
between reality and fantasy. Are those five-dollar cage-free eggs really worth
it? Is that organic banana really any better for your body? Or for the environment? Are the cows happier if they are grass-fed? Or is this all just clever
marketing, designed to make us spend more money?

Here's the truth behind the labels:

GREEN FOOD LABELS, DECODED

Label	Worth the Paper It's Printed On?
All Natural	This label only indicates that the product contains no artifi-cial ingredients, no added color, and is "minimally processed." This label is generally a marketing ploy; for example, high-fructose corn syrup, which is created in a factory but is sourced from a natural ingredient (corn), does not constitute an "artificial ingredient" under this label. All natural does not equal organic.
Cage-Free	This egg label indicates the hens are not kept in cages; cage-free birds do not usually have outdoor access.

Label	Worth the Paper It's Printed On?
Domestic	This label indicates the product comes from the country it is being sold in.
Fair Trade Certified	This regulated label assures customers that farmworkers were paid a fair price for their product and child labor wasn't used to produce the product.
Free-Range or Free-Roam	Animals are not confined to a cage and have access to the outdoors. This label can be misleading. Animals can still be packed tightly and often rarely choose to venture outside because they are scared.
Grass-Fed	This label indicates the cows were fed a more natural grass- or hay-based diet, as opposed to a corn-based diet.
Imported	This label indicates the product comes from outside the country it is being sold in.
Lightly Sweetened	This label is not regulated; "lightly sweetened" does not mean the product is low in sugar.
Local	The "local" label is not regulated, but it generally indicates the product was grown or produced close to the location it is sold in.
Made with Whole Grains	This label indicates that one of the grains in the product is a whole grain; the majority of the grains could be refined grains.
No Added Sugars	This label indicates the product contains no additional sugar or syrups; the product may include natural sugar from fruit or sugar from lactose, for example.
No Antibiotics	This label can be used on cow or chicken products when the producer can supply documentation that the animal was not given antibiotics.
No Hormones Added / Hormone Free	This label indicates the cow was not given any hormones. Hormones cannot legally be given to pigs, chickens, or turkeys.
Non-GMO	Foods with non-GMO on the label indicate the product contains no genetically modified organisms, which are plants or animals whose DNA has been altered. There are no studies that clearly indicate that GMO products are safe for long-term consumption.
Organic	Foods with the organic label contain at least 95 percent organic ingredients. For more information on organic products, see Organic Versus Conventional on page 152.

Label	Worth the Paper It's Printed On?
Trans Fat Free	Before believing this label, check the ingredients list. Products can be labeled as "Trans Fat Free" if they contain less than 0.5 gram of trans fat; double-check that there are no partially hydrogenated or hydrogenated oils in the ingredients list.
Vegetarian-Fed	This label, often found on egg cartons, indicates the animal was fed a vegetarian diet with no animal by-products.
With Added Fiber	Naturally occurring fiber (from fruits, vegetables, or whole grains, for example) has more healthy benefits than artificially added fiber. Check the ingredients for inulin, polydextrose, fructan, chicory extract/fiber/root fiber, fructooligosaccharide, pectin, cellulose, and oligosaccharide, which are all forms of artificially added fiber.

ORGANIC VERSUS CONVENTIONAL

"Organic" is a description for how food is grown, handled, and processed. Farmers who produce organic fruits and vegetables and meat cannot use conventional farming methods, such as pesticides, synthetic fertilizers, or fertilizers created from sewage sludge. Organic products cannot contain GMOs. Animals raised for meat, poultry, eggs, and dairy products cannot be fed antibiotics or growth hormones.

Furthermore, organic meat cannot be treated with ionizing radiation. A treatment process applied to some conventional meat and poultry, food irradiation damages the DNA of microorganisms, bacteria, viruses, and bugs that may be present in the treated food. However, the process may mask food spoilage that occurred prior to irradiation and cause chemical changes in the food that are harmful when consumed. While there is no clear evidence that food irradiation is definitely dangerous to the consumer, there are also no long-term studies that prove the process's safety. And, again, why take that chance? I don't know about you, but I'd rather err on the side of caution when it comes to the food I put in my body.

The following table summarizes the difference between organic and conventional produce, eggs, meat, and dairy. Although "organic" always means fewer chemicals, it does not *always* mean the animals involved in food production are treated more humanely.

ORGANIC AND CONVENTIONAL METHODS

Organic Produce	Conventional Produce
Treating produce with pesticides, fungicides, insecticides, herbicides, antimicrobials, and rodenticides is not permitted; natural methods are used instead.	Farmers may spray produce with pesticides, fungicides, insecticides, herbicides, antimicrobials, and rodenticides.
Organic Eggs	**Conventional Eggs**
Hens must be fed organic feed. Feed cannot contain pesticides, synthetic fertilizers, animal by-products, or GMOs.	Hens are fed conventional feed, which can contain pesticides, synthetic fertilizers, animal by-products, or GMOs.
Hens can only be given antibiotics if there is an infectious disease outbreak.	Healthy hens can be given antibiotics preemptively.
Hens cannot be raised in cages and must have "access to the outdoors," although this doesn't mean the animals venture outside.	Hens can be raised in cages. The typical conventional cage at a factory egg farm is 67 square inches—less than a sheet of paper.[21]
No forced molting. Hens are allowed to molt naturally.	Forced molting is permitted. The process involves restricting food, water, and/or light to encourage hens to shed their feathers and cease egg production, which results in improved egg quality when the molt is over.
Beak trimming/debeaking is permitted. Farmers snip the ends of hens' beaks to control cannibalism and aggressive behavior. The procedure can be painful for the hen.	Beak trimming is permitted.
Male chicks of egg-laying hens are discarded (usually through the use of lethal gas).	Male chicks of egg-laying hens are discarded.

Organic Meat and Dairy	Conventional Meat and Dairy
Animals cannot be fed animal by-products, antibiotics, or sewage sludge. Feed must be organic. Disease is prevented through natural methods; however, antibiotics may be given for serious outbreaks of infectious disease. While on antibiotics, and for a time period after treatment stops, the animal cannot be sold as organic.	Animals can be fed animal by-products (meaning beef-cow feed can contain pig and chicken by-products); the only exception is that cows cannot be directly fed cow by-products. Feed can also contain antibiotics and sewage sludge.
No growth hormones can be given to any livestock.	Dairy and beef cows can be given growth hormones; pigs and poultry cannot.
Total confinement of all animals is prohibited. All animals must have access to the outdoors all year. Ruminant animals (goats, sheep, and cows) must also have "access to pasture" during grazing season.	Animals may be housed entirely indoors.
Organic regulations do not specifically regulate how animals are slaughtered.	While many states have humane slaughter laws, violations are usually considered merely misdemeanors.
Meat cannot be treated with ionizing radiation.	Meat can be treated with ionizing radiation.

There are three categories of organic foods:

- "100 percent organic": These foods cannot contain any nonorganic ingredients.
- "Organic": Foods under this label contain 95 percent organic ingredients. The remaining 5 percent can be conventional ingredients, but cannot contain growth hormones.
- "Made with organic ingredients": This label indicates the food contains at least 70 percent organic ingredients; the remaining portion can be conventionally produced.

Through an official seal, the government makes it easy to sort out the organic labeling system. If the product contains this seal, you know the food is certified to be at least 95 percent organic.

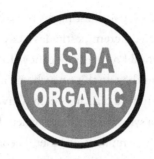

To ensure that farmers and producers comply with strict organic standards, they must be inspected and certified by the government before they can place the organic label on their foods. As you've probably noticed at the grocery store, organic produce and products usually cost more than their conventional counterparts. One reason is the organic certification process itself, which can be very costly for food producers. Another cause of this price discrepancy is that organic farmers do not receive as many subsidies as conventional farmers do. The ingredients in an organic product, such as baking mix, cost more than a conventionally produced "real food" baking mix; this extra cost simply must be passed down to the consumer.

It's tempting to skip the organic goods and buy conventional, especially if money is tight, and it's already a struggle to buy healthy groceries. I've been there—standing in front of a display of apples, holding an organic and conventional fruit in each hand and trying to decide if the organic apple is really worth it. But here's some food for thought: although conventional food is cheaper at checkout, we end up paying for conventional farming in other ways. The first and most obvious way we "pay" for conventional products is through long-term health consequences. Conventional produce contains and is coated in herbicides, pesticides, and antimicrobials; no matter how well you wash a conventional apple, you can't remove the residue of these chemicals from the fleshy part that you eat. While eating one conventional apple clearly doesn't make you keel over and vomit, the impact of these chemicals on your body adds up over time. After all, if a chemical can kill a pest, why wouldn't it harm your body, too? These chemicals are *designed* to do harm.

The Pesticide Action Network estimates that the average American is exposed to ten to thirteen different pesticides a day through their food and drink.[22] The Environmental Protection Agency (EPA) is tasked with regulating such chemicals, but they do this on a chemical-by-chemical basis. It's difficult for the EPA to study and address cumulative impacts and synergistic effects of pesticides (a synergistic effect is when, for example, the chemical effect of one pesticide amplifies another, becoming more toxic when combined). Other nations, particularly those in the European Union, take a more prudent approach. For example, the herbicide atrazine—suspected of being an endocrine disruptor and a possible carcinogen—has been banned in Europe but is still used by American farmers. The cumulative impact of pesticides in an adult's body, or the acute impact of pesticides on a young child or unborn baby, can be devastating. Pesticide exposure has been linked to birth defects, childhood and adult cancer, autism, attention deficit disorder, reproductive issues, development disorders, and neurological diseases.[23]

Pesticides don't just impact health directly through food—these chemicals also contaminate the air we breathe, groundwater we drink, and the soil we walk on. Residential land adjacent to agricultural crops might be the most seriously impacted, especially when pesticides are sprayed or dusted on crops and find their way to surrounding areas; the phenomenon is called pesticide drift. Pesticides also put the farmworkers who tend the land at risk; regular pesticide exposure can lead to acute disease or even death.

When you buy organic, you're buying pesticide-free food. Organic produce is fertilized with manure or compost; insects and rodents are contained through chemical-free methods, such as traps; and weeds are controlled by natural methods, including crop rotation, tilling, or hand weeding.

WASH FIRST

If you do choose to eat conventional produce, you can reduce the amount of pesticides you consume by following these simple steps, as suggested by the Environmental Protection Agency:

- **Wash:** Thoroughly wash all fruits and vegetables under running water. Use your hands or a clean, soft brush to scrub the outside of the produce; friction will help remove more of the chemicals than simply soaking the fruit or vegetables. Be sure to wash produce even if you do not plan on eating the skin. When you slice an orange, for example, the knife will transfer pesticides (germs, too) from the outside of the fruit to the fleshy part you consume.
- **Peel and Trim:** The edible skin of fruits and vegetables is a great source of fiber and nutrients. But if it's conventional produce, remove the skin—where the majority of the pesticides lurk. For heads of greens (lettuce, kale, or collard greens, for example), throw away the larger outside leaves that were exposed to the most pesticides. If you're consuming conventional meat, poultry, or fish, remove any fatty deposits, since pesticides tend to concentrate in fat.

Do you need to wash organic produce, too? Yes! Just imagine all the hands and surfaces your produce has touched before you bring it home. Washing produce under warm water can remove potentially harmful bacteria, including salmonella, listeria, and E. coli.

Second, there are long-term environmental costs associated with conventional farming. More than one billion pounds of pesticides are used on American farms, forests, lawns, and golf courses each year; these chemicals seep into bodies of water, penetrate the soil, and contaminate the air we breathe. Organic farming is better for the immediate environment, because it reduces air, water, and soil pollution; conserves water; combats soil erosion (due to organic farming's practice of maintaining generally thicker topsoil and higher organic content in the soil); and increases soil vitality. Organic farming also generally uses less energy than conventional methods. While proponents of pesticides argue that the chemicals increase crop yields, making food less expensive, this is a short-term fix. Studies show that pesticides damage soil's vitality, reducing yields over time. Furthermore, pesticide resistance is rapidly increasing, making plants more susceptible to attack by new diseases and pests.

ORGANIC'S IMMEDIATE IMPACT

A 2006 study of elementary school children revealed that switching to an organic diet reduced the amount of organophosphorus pesticides (an insecticide that is suspected of having adverse effects on the neurobehavioral development of fetuses and children) present in the children's urine. Instead of eating conventional fruit and vegetables, juices, and wheat- and corn-based items such as pasta and cereal, the children feasted on similar organic options. Levels of organophosphorus pesticides dropped immediately and then tapered off to a "nondetect" level after two weeks on the new organic diet, proving that an organic diet provides immediate and dramatic protection against pesticide exposure in food.[24]

There are other long-term health and environmental costs from conventional farming methods, as well. When conventionally raised livestock, dairy-producing animals, and egg-laying hens are given antibiotics and growth hormones, the final product, the one on your plate, contains trace amounts of these drugs. Amazingly, the livestock industry gives antibiotics to *healthy* conventionally raised animals to prevent disease and ensure they grow as large as possible, as fast as possible. As much as 70 percent of antibiotics used in America are distributed to cattle, chickens, pigs, and other livestock, not sick people.[25] In 2011, the FDA acknowledged this practice was creating a public-health crisis by contributing to the evolution of multidrug-resistant bacteria that can infect humans.

Conventional livestock can also be fed the flesh of other animals or animals of their own species—yes, really! That means that egg-laying conventional hens feast on a mix that contains chicken flesh, upping the risk for disease. Due to the outbreak of mad cow disease, cattle cannot be re-fed cattle, but they can be fed chicken that were fed cattle, a nasty little loophole.

Often, people assume that organic produce and products contain more nutrients than their conventional counterparts; this has not been proven. However, it's not really about what organic has *more* of—it's what it has *less* of. No pesticides, no GMOs, no antibiotics, no growth hormones, no food irradiation. Just natural food.

People also often assume that organic food is going to be terribly expensive when compared to conventional products, but if you shop wisely, the cost differential between conventional and organic really isn't *that* much (especially considering the tremendous benefits of eating organic!). Thankfully, as the demand for organic foods increases, the cost difference between organic and conventional will become even smaller.

One way to find inexpensive organic produce is to shop at local farmers' markets or join a community supported agriculture (CSA) group (for more information about local options, check out pages 162–66). If you're buying organic at the grocery store, purchase only in-season produce, which is always cheaper than imported foods. Many warehouse clubs, such as Costco, offer a variety of organic options in bulk. If you're a gardener, consider switching to organic methods and growing your own fruits and vegetables.

If you cannot buy 100 percent organic, you can greatly reduce your pesticide exposure by avoiding the so-called Dirty Dozen, a list of twelve conventionally grown fruits and vegetables that are the most contaminated. These are the most important to buy organic, according to the Environmental Working Group. Similarly, the EWG has prepared a list of the Clean Fifteen, which are the least contaminated. The Dirty Dozen and Clean Fifteen lists following can help you cost-effectively reduce your overall pesticide exposure.

SHOP SMART: THE MOST AND LEAST
CONTAMINATED PRODUCTS

Dirty Dozen (Buy Organic)	Clean Fifteen (Lowest in Pesticides)
Apples	Onions
Celery	Sweet corn
Strawberries	Pineapples
Peaches	Avocado
Spinach	Asparagus
Nectarines, imported	Sweet peas
Grapes, imported	Mangoes
Sweet bell peppers	Eggplant
White potatoes	Domestic cantaloupe
Domestic blueberries	Kiwi
Lettuce	Cabbage
Kale/Collard greens	Watermelon
	Sweet potatoes
	Grapefruit
	Mushrooms

Source: Environmental Working Group, 2011

Don't let the Dirty Dozen list scare you away from buying fruits and vegetables. It's more important to eat *any* fruit or vegetable—conventional or not—rather than skip plants entirely.

Is organic the be-all and end-all? Well, not to further confuse the issue, but no! The tricky thing is that organic is not *always* better for the environment. Organic blueberries from Chile were overnighted to your supermarket on a fuel-guzzling airplane. This is where the local versus organic debate comes in; this topic is explored more on page 162. Organic is not necessarily better for the animals, either, as shown in the Organic and Conventional Methods comparison on page 153.

Body wash made from all-natural ingredients can be expensive. Dilute it with equal parts water to stretch your dollar.

Healthy Tipping Point Success Story: Jenna, 26, Illinois

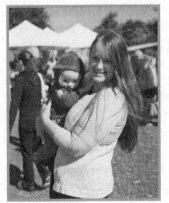

My diet was very typical for an American. The nutrition label was king, and I wouldn't buy anything without checking the amount of saturated fat and the amount of protein. (I wanted lots of protein and the least amount of saturated fat possible.) I never, ever checked the list of ingredients because I thought the important information was found in the numbers: grams, calories, percentages.

About five years ago, my dad, a full-time farmer, switched from growing conventional onions to organic farming exclusively, and my interest in where my food came from grew. I found that I wasn't concerned only with the food's numbers or how it tasted, I wanted to know how it was grown, and who was doing the growing, and I wanted it as fresh as possible. I felt overwhelmed at first, but the first step was going to the farmers' market. At first, I didn't ask any questions of the growers, but then I learned it's okay to question. Now, when I approach the stand I ask, "Is this conventional or organic?" and "You didn't spray fertilizer, but did you *use* fertilizer?" I visited one organic farmer often enough that he started giving me a returning customer discount!

I used to treat vegetables as an icky side dish to force down before I got to the good stuff, but each time I visited the market, I was so excited about the offerings that I came home with overflowing bags of tomatoes, peppers, summer squash, and berries that needed to be used up. Vegetables went from the side of my plate to being the star of the show!

Though it was difficult to get up for the market each Saturday, I found myself looking forward to my early-morning Saturday shopping ritual. When winter came, and the markets closed, I felt a bit lost. By using sites like Local Harvest (www.localharvest.org), I was able to find a community-supported agriculture group that continued through the winter. I paid ahead of time, and a box was dropped off on the back porch of a local church every two weeks. This supplied my family with apples, potatoes, onions, squash, and other fresh, local produce through the winter months. Eventually, we hope to live in a place where we can have a garden. Fruits and vegetables have become something to look forward to, and I admit there are days when I just can't get enough.

MILES ON THE PLATE

Many people choose to eat organic foods for the environmental benefits, but if your organic blueberries come from Chile or even if your organic apples come from the other side of America, there is another significant environmental cost: food miles. Food miles are a measurement of the distance a food product must travel between where it is grown to where it is sold. With an increased demand for a greater variety of foods, as well as an increased demand for all types of produce to be available year round, food miles have skyrocketed in recent years:

- The West Coast supplies 75 percent of the apples sold in New York City.
- In 2007, it was estimated that food products traveled 25 percent farther from farm to plate than in 1980.

- The typical meal in America includes, on average, ingredients from at least five foreign countries. [26]

Increasing food miles means increasing fossil fuel emissions. Whether transported by truck, plane, or ship, moving food over thousands of miles pumps a significant quantity of carbon emissions into the atmosphere, impacts our air quality and health, and contributes to larger environmental issues such as global warming. It's worth noting that there are other issues at play beyond food miles; for many foods, the manufacturing or growing process produces far more carbon emissions than transporting the goods thousands of miles (especially if the produce is not organic and the carbon emissions created from the production of pesticides and fertilizers are counted). Also, just because a food didn't travel far to arrive at your grocer doesn't mean it's environmentally greener. The amount of fossil fuels involved in importing tomatoes, for example, might be less than the amount associated with growing tomatoes locally in a hothouse.

While there are some exceptions to the food-mile philosophy, it's safe to say that, in general, importing food products has a negative environmental impact. The issue of food miles should certainly be considered when selecting produce.

Opting for local products and produce, when available, reduces the carbon footprint of your meal. There are other advantages to buying local— it's good for the regional economy; supports small, family-owned farms; and preserves open space. Local food is also healthier and tastier. A fruit imported from another country is harvested; stored; cleaned; processed; transported via truck, air, or sea; and driven to your grocer. What you think of as fresh produce might not be that fresh at all. Local produce may contain more nutrients than imported produce since the local option is often consumed closer to the harvest date. Fresher is better, for so many reasons!

THE LONGER YOU WAIT, THE MORE YOU LOSE

One study revealed that green beans lose 45 percent of their nutrients in the eleven to fifteen days between harvest, transport, sale, and at-home preparation. Broccoli loses 25 percent of its nutrients in the same time span.[27]

Local and organic produce are the best option, but not everyone has access to a variety of fresh local produce year round. The global food system is very large and complex, and it's not always black and white; the local versus imported issue can become very murky. Are conventional but local blueberries better for the planet and your health than imported but organic blueberries? Maybe . . . or maybe not. After all, while the conventional blueberries contain trace amounts of pesticides and other chemicals, they may be fresher and thus contain more nutrients than the potentially older organic blueberries. The carbon emissions created by shipping the organic blueberries from a foreign country may or may not be more than the emissions created by manufacturing pesticides for the conventional but local berries.

Truthfully, in our global economy, there is no perfect way to grocery shop for the environment, your health, and your wallet. And being perfect isn't a realistic goal of the green movement, anyway; more than anything, it's about simply being a conscious consumer and making better choices when feasible. Small efforts—for your health and the environment—really do add up, both personally and globally.

Healthy, organic, and sustainable eating has a bad reputation as being pricey and budget-busting. Here are five ways to become a more conscious and more budget-savvy grocery shopper:

- **Shop in season:** You can get blueberries in Wisconsin in the middle of November, but at what cost? Buying produce that is out of season is unsustainable because of high food miles, and in-season produce is often fresher, cheaper, and (more often than not) locally or regionally grown. A little bonus: buying in-season produce will also ensure you eat a greater variety of fruits and vegetables in the course of a year!

One way to ensure you buy in season is to skip making strict grocery lists that call for specific types of produce. For example, instead of writing, "I need kale, broccoli, butternut squash, oranges, and kiwi," plan to buy general categories of fruits and veggies, such as "I need a few green veggies and several pieces of whole fruit." Then, when you get to the store, check to see which items are advertised as being on sale (a sign that a crop is in season). Produce that is prominently displayed is also typically in season.

In-season fruits and veggies will vary greatly by your location. For more information, check out Web sites such as Sustainable Table (www.sustainabletable.org), which offer lists of in-season produce by state.

- **Shop at a farmers' market:** Regularly shopping at a farmers' market, when available, is a great way to interact with and support local farmers and businesspeople. Most farmers' markets offer a variety of foods, not just produce, at prices that are comparable to or less than grocery store prices. Many markets offer organic options as well. But be warned—just because it's at a farmers' market doesn't mean it's local. If you see bananas in New Hampshire in July, they were probably imported to the market. Farmers at the market usually enjoy talking to customers about their foods and growing practices, so feel free to ask questions.

- **Join a CSA:** Consider joining a community-supported agriculture (CSA) network, which connects local farmers and local consumers. CSA members receive a box of fresh fruits and vegetables each week. CSAs cost approximately fifteen to thirty dollars a week for four to six months, and each weekly box usually includes six to ten different fruits and veggies. For an additional fee, many CSAs will even deliver the box directly to a member's front door! Some CSAs have expanded to offer members other foods, such as locally produced eggs, bread, meat, or poultry. CSA products are typically certified organic or, at the very least, produced using organic methods.

CSAs are an amazing way to support local farmers, encourage sustainable and organic agriculture, and save money and reduce grocery shopping time—all while eating healthy, nutritious foods. Local Harvest (www.localharvest.org) offers a database of more than 4,000 American CSAs.

> Line produce drawers with organic paper towels; they'll absorb excess moisture and delay rot in fruits and vegetables. Replace the papers after every shopping trip.

- **Petition your grocery store:** If you feel your neighborhood grocery store is lacking local options, ask the manager to specifically stock a variety of local choices. Most grocery stores are very open to customer requests and will work hard to fill them.
- **Eat more meatless meals:** Plant-based eaters choose to eat the way they do for a variety of reasons, and for many, the most compelling reason is their own health. A diet rich in plants and low in meat and sweets is naturally higher in nutrients and lower in saturated fat and cholesterol, which contributes to vitality in the short and long terms. But there are other reasons to eat more plants and less meat, and these reasons are often just as (or even more) compelling.

At the grocery store, it's easy to forget that meat was once a living, breathing animal. It's difficult to imagine a cow or chicken when you're staring at row after row of perfectly uniform, shrink-wrapped meat. For most of us, meat has ceased to be an animal product—it's just simply a food. But the reality, of course, is that bacon is pig, hot wings are chickens, and hamburgers are cows, and these animals have to be born, raised, and slaughtered before their products appear neatly wrapped in your grocer's refrigerator case.

EAT YOUR DOG?

Here's some food for thought: why do you eat some animals, but not others? Most Westerners are horrified at the thought of eating a cat, dog, or horse (a practice common in other areas of the world), but don't think twice about eating a cow, pig, or chicken. Livestock animals are just as (if not more) intelligent than domesticated pets and are capable of a similar range of emotions. Really, the only difference between a pig and a dog is that one has earned the cultural distinction of man's best friend, and the other is destined for our dinner plate.

Think about all the meat, dairy, and eggs that are served in American homes and restaurants each day. These animal products must come from *somewhere,* and odds are the original owner of those hot wings didn't live on an idyllic country farm with wide-open pastures—as a matter of fact, that chicken might have never even seen daylight. Most of our meat comes from large-scale factory farms, where animals are viewed as a bottom line, not as a living creature. Conditions are often cruel and uncomfortable; giving animals space, freedom, and high-quality feed negatively impacts profit. If you want to make a lot of meat, and you want to do it cheaply, you have to cut corners, and the creatures that suffer the most end up on your plate. Animals receive cheap, conventional feed packed with corn, animal by-products, antibiotics, growth hormones, GMOs, and a variety of other unnatural ingredients, depending on the type of animal. Conventional feed can contribute to new types of diseases, such as those caused by outbreaks of previously unknown E. coli strains, and impacts on a variety of health issues in the "end users"—humans.

Factory-scale slaughtering is no better. The majority of beef in all of

America is slaughtered at one of thirteen massive slaughterhouse operations.[28] Just imagine what would happen if a contagious disease erupted at one of these major slaughterhouses! And the government lacks the teeth to fully protect consumers; while the USDA once held the power to shut down plants that repeatedly failed salmonella and E. coli testing, major meat and poultry associations went to court to have this power stripped away. The FDA, tasked with completing food safety inspections, only conducted 9,164 inspections in 2006—down from more than 50,000 in 1972.[29]

The cheap hamburger at the grocery store; the four-dollar chicken sandwich from a chain restaurant; the sausage sandwiches at the baseball game—these animal products most likely did not come from a quaint family-owned farm. The animals that died for your meal were raised in factories, and they were slaughtered in factories.

Yes—there are family-owned farms all over the country that are directed by caring men and women who strive to keep their animals healthy and happy. These small-scale farmers should not be condemned. But the cold, hard truth is that the United States could not possibly produce such staggering quantities of meat and poultry without doing most of the raising and slaughtering on a factory scale.

In addition to these animal cruelty issues and human health risks, factory farming extracts a major environmental price. Livestock production directly or indirectly takes up more than 30 percent of our world's non-ice land. There are roughly 15,500 concentrated animal feeding operations (CAFOs) in the United States; imagine large swatches of unvegetated land packed with more than 1,000 beef cattle, 30,000 broiler chickens, or 125,000 egg-laying chickens. Imagine the stink of feces from all these animals. Imagine how this contamination impacts the surrounding surface water and groundwater. The Environmental Protection Agency estimates that 75 percent of our nation's water-quality problems are a direct result of agriculture (and most of our agriculture is indirectly or directly associated with livestock production).[30] CAFOs also pollute the air; it's estimated that livestock production creates 20 percent of global greenhouse gas emissions and 7 percent of emissions in America.[31] As a result, people who live within a few miles of a CAFO report a host of health issues, including nausea, eye irritation, asthma, and weakness.

Did you know that the majority of corn and soy grown in the world feeds cattle, pigs, and chickens—not people? Using so much corn and soy on animals is essentially a waste; two to five times more grain is required to produce the same amount of calories consumed by eating livestock as through direct food consumption.[32]

> Ditch the deli meat—make sandwiches with hummus, nut butter, or veggie burger patties.

Feeding our world's thirst for meat is expensive: morally, economically, and environmentally. But you can make a difference, and you don't even have to give up meat. Simply eat *less* meat and *more* plants—this is about finding balance on your plate, not restricting a certain food. Eating more plants is cheaper at checkout and helps improve conditions in factory farms and slaughterhouses by reducing the demand for meat. Vegetarian dining is also much, much more environmentally friendly. Amazingly, if every American reduced their meat consumption by 20 percent, it would be like everyone trading in their gas-guzzling sedan for an environmentally friendly hybrid, according to research done by the University of Chicago.[33]

If you do choose to consume meat, reach for more nutritional *and* sustainable options. Select salmon, tuna, lean beef or turkey, or chicken instead of fatty hamburger meat. While the organic label doesn't necessarily guarantee the animals were treated any more humanely (see pages 152–56 for more information), organic meat production doesn't exact the same horrendous toll on the environment as conventional methods. You can also visit a local farmers' market to search out local meat producers that operate on a smaller scale and treat the animals with greater respect. And yes—this does mean your meat will be more expensive pound for pound, but if you're eating more meatless meals, the cost difference will equal out.

READ, WATCH, AND EAT

Want to learn more about the ramifications of our complex global food economy, and how you can make healthier and more environmentally conscious choices? Check out these intriguing and educational books and movies for more information.

BOOKS

Fast Food Nation, Eric Schlosser (Harper Perennial, 2005)
The Omnivore's Dilemma, Michael Pollan (Penguin, 2007)
Animal, Vegetable, Miracle, Barbara Kingsolver (Harper Perennial, 2008)
In Defense of Food, Michael Pollan (Penguin, 2009)
Eating Animals, Jonathan Safran Foer (Back Bay Books, 2010)

MOVIES

King Corn (2007)
The World According to Monsanto (2008)
Food Inc. (2008)
FoodMatters (2008)
Tapped (2009)
Forks Over Knives (2011)

Seven

HEALTHY EATING IN PRACTICE

age-free, vitamin B, protein powders—oh my! Food really is about more than taste; healthy eating becomes a complicated mix of science, budget, emotions, and ethics. How these issues boil down and impact your daily eating is a truly personal decision, and there is certainly no right or wrong way to eat real food.

In driver's ed class, the instructors droned on and on about turning signals and braking speeds and right-of-ways, but it really meant nothing until you actually sat behind the wheel. This section focuses on how to put your new food knowledge into practice at the store, on the go, at work, in the kitchen, and dining out in restaurants. And remember—it's not about being the perfect eater. It's about making small choices that add up to a balanced diet that makes you feel strong and happy.

Healthy Out and About

Most of us eat several meals a week—if not a meal a day—out at a restaurant, a coffee shop, or from a food truck. Diet books preach that it's impossible to eat out and eat healthy; the reality is that it's not difficult, as long as you pay attention to cooking methods and portion size.

Avoid foods that are described as fried (including pan-fried or deep-fried), au gratin, battered, basted, or breaded. Skip dishes that include cream sauce (including Alfredo sauce, hollandaise, or vodka sauce). While cream sauces aren't inherently unhealthy, it's easy to overdo it with restaurant-size portions. If you're eating meat, choose entrees that are described as baked, broiled, grilled, poached, roasted, or steamed. Consider becoming a "restaurant vegetarian" and order meatless choices when dining out—they are usually healthier *and* cheaper than their meat counterparts.

Don't be afraid to ask for substitutions or modifications. If you are polite to the server (and tip well), he or she won't mind a special request. Ask if you can swap the side of fries or mashed potatoes for steamed veggies, a side salad, or a fruit salad. While most restaurants pre-prepare their vegetables with a butter sauce, the greens are still healthier than fries. At Chinese or Thai restaurants, ask for brown rice instead of white. At pizzerias, order thin crust and load up on the vegetables—not the meat. You can also request a lighter sprinkle of cheese.

Salads are a great option at a restaurant, as long as the salad isn't loaded down with cheese, croutons, tortilla strips, and creamy dressing. Request these items on the side, so you can control how much goes onto your salad, or skip them altogether. Ask for vinaigrette dressing or olive oil and vinegar. Get the salad dressing, and all other condiments, on the side so you can control the portion. Mayonnaise isn't intrinsically bad; it's only unhealthy when you eat a quarter cup on a sandwich!

> Enjoy one "extra" when dining out—bread, appetizer, or dessert—not all three.

You'll also want to pay attention to portion control, because restaurants tend to serve up dishes that are really two, three, or four servings. Splitting an entree with your dining companion or immediately boxing up half is a great way to ensure you don't overeat. Only eat one extra in addition to your entree—such as a bread roll, an appetizer, or a dessert.

Last, check out the restaurant's Web site before dining out. Many chains and larger restaurants provide the nutritional information for their foods online. This can help you make healthier and more balanced decisions when you sit down to eat.

Healthy at the Store

Did you know that the average American hits the grocery store two times a week? Did you know the average American opens their fridge, stares despondently, and announces, "There's nothing to eat!" at least four times a week?

All right, that last statistic is completely fabricated. But it's certainly true that most people struggle to turn groceries into healthy meals, open produce drawers and find untouched rotting veggies, and end up ordering takeout even though their pantry is stocked. The secret to wonderful, healthy meals isn't necessarily buying *more* food—it's buying the *healthiest* foods in *recipe-friendly combinations*.

HEALTHY BUYING GUIDE

First, we'll tackle buying the healthiest foods. The buying guide below is an extensive, but not exhaustive, list of healthy foods available at most grocery stores and farmers' markets.

GENERAL HEALTHY BUYING GUIDE

Pantry Items	Special Notes
Balsamic vinegar	
Barley	For grain preparation tips, see page 218.
BBQ sauce	Check the label for high-fructose corn syrup (HFCS) and artificial sweeteners.

Pantry Items	Special Notes
Bread crumbs or panko crumbs	Check the ingredients list for hydrogenated oils.
Brown rice	For grain preparation tips, see page 218.
Bulgar	For grain preparation tips, see page 218.
Canned artichokes	Look for artichokes packed in water, not oil.
Canned beans (pinto, kidney, chickpea, navy, black beans, white beans)	Buy several cans of chickpeas and use them in home-made hummus (see the recipe for Spinach Hummus on page 231).
Canned soup	Check the ingredients list for HFCS and MSG. Opt for low-sodium options.
Capers	Capers are an excellent and flavorful addition to salads.
Condiments—ketchup, mustard, for example	Check the ingredients list for HFCS and artificial colors.
Flour (whole wheat, white, spelt, or buckwheat are popular choices)	You can't substitute whole wheat or other types of minimally processed flour for white flour without making adjustments. Check online for recipe modifications for different flour types. Store flour in a tightly sealed container in the freezer.
Granulated sugar and brown sugar	
Herbs and spices	There are many different herbs and spices, but the most versatile ones include fresh parsley (add to Italian-flavored dishes); fresh cilantro (add to Latin-inspired dishes); fresh basil (delicious in salads); minced garlic; fresh ginger (steep to make tea, see page 149); curry powder; ground cinnamon; chili powder; and pepper and salt.
Jarred salsa	
Lentils (red, green, or brown) or split peas	
Millet	For grain preparation tips, see page 219.
Nut butters (peanut butter, almond butter, sunflower butter, tahini butter)	Buy natural nut butters and avoid reduced-fat brands. Refrigerate after opening. If the oil and nuts in natural nut butters separate, simply stir thoroughly.
Nutritional yeast	As a flavoring for vegetables or in a sauce.

Pantry Items	Special Notes
Nuts and seeds (cashews, pecans, almonds, walnuts, sunflower seeds)	
Oils (extra-virgin olive, canola, peanut)	
Old-fashioned oatmeal	Skip the flavored packets, which are expensive and loaded with sugar and fake foods. These flavors are easy to create at home with your own real-food ingredients (for example, add sliced apples and cinnamon to cooked oatmeal).
Pure maple syrup	
Quinoa	For grain preparation tips, see page 219.
Salad dressing	Opt for oil-based, not cream-based, dressings, and check the ingredients list for artificial flavors or colors and HFCS. Alternatively, create your own dressings; see pages 223–24 for recipes.
Tomato sauce	Check the label for HFCS.
Vegetable broth	Buy low-sodium when possible.
Whole-grain bread	
Whole-grain cereals	Look for cereals that have less than 10 grams of sugar per serving and are fortified with vitamin B_{12}.
Whole-grain pasta	
Whole-grain tortillas	Check the ingredients list for hydrogenated oil (trans fat) and lard.
Whole wheat crackers	
Whole wheat pancake / biscuit mix	
Wild rice	For grain preparation tips, see page 219.
Yeast	
Refrigerated Protein and Dairy Items	Special Notes
Cheese	Consume in moderation.
Eggs	Opt for organic and cage free when possible (for more on egg carton labeling, see page 150).

Refrigerated Protein and Dairy Items	Special Notes
Extra-firm fortified tofu	See page 189 for instructions on baking tofu.
Faux meat alternatives	
Fish and seafood	Opt for sustainable options, as described on the Natural Resources Defense Council's Web site (http://www.nrdc.org/oceans/seafoodguide).
Free-range organic poultry	Consume in moderation.
Grass-fed organic beef	Consume in moderation.
Hummus	
Low-fat or skim milk or milk alternatives	See page 143 for a list of milk alternatives.
Organic yogurt	It's important to buy organic yogurt because it offers more strains of digestive-friendly probiotics than conventional yogurt. Greek yogurt packs an extra protein punch, too. Check the ingredients list for HFCS and artificial sweeteners.
Tempeh	

Non-Alcoholic Beverages	Special Notes
Coconut water	Touted as nature's alternative to sports energy drinks, coconut water is a source of electrolytes and potassium and helps rehydrate the body after a sweaty workout.
Coffee	The jury is still out on coffee: some say it's healthy, others argue that java is harmful. The effects of coffee largely boil down to how much you consume, and what you add to it. Limit it to one cup a day and flavor your brew with organic milk or milk alternatives and real sugar, agave nectar, honey, or stevia. Skip the artificial flavors and sweeteners. Also, opt for organic and fair-trade coffee.
Green tea	Green tea is much healthier than coffee. Packed with antioxidants, new research suggests green tea can increase bone mineral density.[34]

Non-Alcoholic Beverages	Special Notes
Juices	Juices get a bad rap because some juices have added sugar and artificial colors. Juice lacks the fiber found in whole fruit. Also, if you sip on juice all day long, you're potentially drinking a lot of extra calories. However, 100 percent juice has its place. A small cup of orange juice in the morning is a nice alternative if you're too rushed to sit down and eat a whole fruit. It's also a good snack if you're searching for a healthy option on the road or at the airport.
Teeccino herbal coffee	Teecino brews and tastes like your regular cup of coffee, but it's actually made from herbs, grains, fruits, and nuts—thus, caffeine-free "coffee."
Water	Aim to drink half of your weight in pounds in ounces of water each day. If you eat many plants (which naturally contain water), you may need less. If you exercise, you may need more.
Yerba maté	Yerba maté is a coffeelike beverage that is derived from the leaves of rainforest holly trees. It's often touted as having the strength of coffee and the health benefits of tea.

Freezer Items	Special Notes
Frozen fruits for smoothies	Try strawberries, peaches, or blueberries.
Frozen vegetables	Peas, corn, or broccoli are good veggie staples.
Veggie burger patties	
Whole wheat pizza dough, whole wheat frozen veggie pizzas	For pizza dough recipes, see the ½ and ½ Pizza Dough recipe on page 209.

Produce Items	Special Notes
Note: It is impractical to list every type of produce available at the grocery store, so only the most common choices are listed. In order to eat a healthy, plant-based diet, you'll need to grocery shop once a week to stock up on fresh produce. Since many people struggle to fit fruits and vegetables into their diet, the Special Notes section includes buying and preparation tips. And remember—it's better for your health, the environment, and your wallet to shop in season, buy organic, and support local farmers.	
Apples	An apple's nutrients lie mainly within the skin, so don't peel! For a healthy dessert option, try the Baked Apples recipe on page 230.

Produce Items	Special Notes
Asparagus	The end of an asparagus spear is tough and unpalatable. Bend the spear in half; it will naturally break along the point the spear transitions from tough to tender.
Avocados	Ripe avocados will give slightly when squeezed; buy firm fruit if you plan to eat it in a few days.
Bananas	For thicker, creamier smoothies, add frozen banana slices. It's best to freeze a banana after the skin has browned, and the fruit is at its sweetest. Just remember to peel and slice before placing in freezer-safe plastic bags.
Beets	Beets' powerful phytonutrient, betalain, is easily diminished by high heat. To protect the beet, do not remove the skin and steam for only 15–20 minutes; do not overcook. Once a fork can be inserted, the beet is done. Rub with a paper towel to remove the skin.
Bell peppers (green, red, yellow)	Remove the top of the pepper and the inner seeds. Stuff with cooked brown rice, chopped tomatoes, and drained and rinsed kidney beans. Top with cheese. Bake at 350 degrees for 30 minutes.
Berries	To prevent spoilage, store in the fridge and check daily for freshness. Removing one moldy berry will help prevent the spread of this produce ruiner.
Bok choy	Baby bok choy is light and sweet; add it to stir-fry dishes.
Broccoli	Just ½ cup of broccoli has 100 percent of the recommended daily intake of vitamins A and C. Try the Simple Roasted Broccoli (page 225).
Cabbage	To maximize the nutrients in cabbage, steam until the vegetable just begins to soften, but not past that point.
Carrots	Larger carrots are generally sweeter than smaller ones. Don't buy those bags labeled "baby carrots"; they are simply larger carrots cut into small sizes for convenience's sake, and they provide no unique health benefits.

Produce Items	Special Notes
Cauliflower	After removing the stem and any leaves, coarsely chop a head of cauliflower; steam; mash; and spice with chopped parsley, salt, and pepper. Drizzle with a bit of olive oil and serve as an alternative to mashed potatoes.
Celery	To keep celery fresh, cut off ends, place in a large tumbler filled with an inch of water, and put in fridge.
Cherries	Select dark and firm (but not hard) cherries.
Citrus (orange, grapefruit)	Don't judge an orange by its cover—nonorganic oranges are often brightly colored because growers inject Citrus Red Number 2 into the fruit skins. Select oranges that are smooth and heavy; those oranges will be juicier.
Collard greens	Packed with vitamins K, A, and C, magnesium, folate, and calcium, collard greens make an excellent side dish—just steam, drain, and drizzle with a little soy sauce.
Corn	Use your fingernail to pop a kernel; if the corn is fresh, a milky substance will leak out.
Cucumbers	Instead of crackers or chips, try dipping cucumbers in hummus or salsa.
Eggplant	If overly ripe, eggplant can taste bitter when baked, grilled, or stir-fried. Cube the eggplant, sprinkle it with salt, and allow it to stand an hour. The salt will draw out the bitter compound through osmosis. Remove extra salt by rinsing under cold water.
Grapes	Choose red over green—red grapes are a good source of anthocyanins, which have anti-inflammatory and antioxidant properties.
Kale	Considered a superfood because of its antioxidant and anti-inflammatory properties.
Kiwi	For an extra fiber boost, eat the skin of the kiwi—yes, really!
Lemons and limes	Start your day off with a cup of warm water and lemon juice. Lemons are an excellent source of the immune-boosting vitamin C and are thought to have a detoxifying effect.

Produce Items	Special Notes
Melon (watermelon, cantaloupe)	Make a fresh salad with watermelon or cantaloupe cubes, fresh basil leaves, and feta cheese.
Mushrooms	Mushrooms act like sponges, so don't soak them before cooking. Simply rinse quickly with water and use a paper towel to rub off any remaining dirt.
Papaya	Purchase papayas with reddish-orange skin that are slightly soft to the touch. Green papayas should not be purchased, but yellowish papayas will ripen at home within several days. For an extra kick, squeeze fresh lemon or lime juice on papaya cubes.
Parsnips	Peel, chop, and drizzle parsnips with a bit of olive oil and salt. Roast at 375 degrees for 35 minutes and serve with ketchup.
Peaches	The darker the peach, the more vitamin A!
Pears	Pears are ready to eat when their skin gives way to gentle pressure. Let pears ripen on the counter, not in the fridge, for the best flavor.
Plums	Don't be afraid of prunes—they're simply dried plums!
Pomegranate	To cut open a pomegranate, slice off ½ inch of the crown (top), which will expose the white membranes. Use a sharp knife to score the outside of the pomegranate along the membrane. Fill a bowl with water and submerge the fruit. Pull apart the sections and use your fingers to pull off the seeds, keeping the fruit underwater to prevent splattering. The membranes will float to the top of the water and the edible seeds will sink to the bottom.
Potatoes	The most nutritious potatoes are also the most colorful. White potatoes are lacking in carotenoids, a pigment with cancer-fighting properties. Sweet, red, or purple potatoes are much more nutritious. Choose small, golf ball–size potatoes over larger ones, since smaller potatoes have a higher skin-to-starch ratio. Potato skin is a great source of fiber and nutrients. Sweet potatoes, in particular, are an excellent source of beta-carotene and vitamin A—just be sure to eat your sweet potato with 3–5 grams of fat because this promotes uptake of these important nutrients. A light drizzle of olive oil does the trick.

Produce Items	Special Notes
Salad greens	Skip iceberg lettuce or other pale leafy choices and go for the darker greens.
Spinach	Add handfuls of spinach to smoothies during the blending process; promise that you won't taste it!
Sprouts	Sprouts are a tasty addition to sandwiches and salads, but people with suppressed immune systems—due to pregnancy or cancer, for example—should skip 'em because bacteria can thrive in raw sprouts.
Squash (yellow, butternut, spaghetti, zucchini)	Swap out the pasta in lasagna for thin slices of yellow squash and zucchini.
Tomatoes	Tomatoes are rich in a carotenoid called lycopene, which is thought to prevent cancer and cardiovascular disease. Organic ketchup delivers three times as much lycopene as nonorganic brands!

Salty Snacks and Desserts	Special Notes
Chocolate and candies	Review the ingredients list for fake foods, such as artificial colors or sweeteners.
Cookies	Review the ingredients list for fake foods, such as artificial colors or sweeteners, and trans fat.
Ice cream	Opt for wholesome ice creams made from the basics—milk, cream, sugar, and natural flavors, like vanilla or chocolate. Alternatively, seek out nondairy choices, including ice cream made from coconut milk or soy milk.
Potato chips and crackers	Check the ingredient lists for fake foods, especially MSG or artificial colors. Select lower-sodium options when possible.

Healthy Tipping Point Success Story: Stephanie, 36, Texas

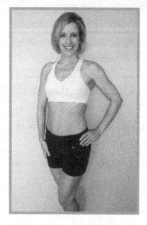

My family was sliding back into unhealthy habits. As a working mom with two kids, picking up fast food or ordering pizza for dinner after a long day sounded much easier than cooking. And although I tried to exercise a few times a week, I realized that I had put on about ten pounds, and my running shoes had been in the back of my closet for two years!

In January 2011, I decided to commit to making healthier lifestyle choices for my entire family. First, I started with the food we ate. We joined a produce co-op to receive local, seasonal, organic produce every other week. I started adding fruits and vegetables into every meal; switched to whole wheat bread, pasta, and rice; and began buying organic dairy and meat. Although convenient, fast food is so processed and unhealthy that we eliminated it completely from our diet. Instead, my husband and I take turns cooking or grilling a few times a week. When we go on road trips, we always pack our own food.

To encourage my kids to actually eat these new, healthy foods, I got them involved in all aspects of eating. I take my daughter to the grocery store so she can help me pick out fresh bananas, avocados, and broccoli. Kids are more willing to eat foods that they help prepare, so I ask my kids to chop lettuce and other soft vegetables with a butter knife while I am cooking. We also keep presliced veggies, fruit, and low-fat cheese in the bottom drawers of the fridge so the kids can help themselves to snacks. Our family also loves to bake. My two-year-old son holds the mixing bowl while my four-year-old daughter pours in the ingredients that I have premeasured. Last year, we even planted a small garden where we grow tomatoes, peppers, and cucumbers. The kids love to eat anything that we have grown in our own backyard.

I also decided to make exercise a priority in my life—not an option. Because I have a husband, career, and two kids that keep me busy, I need time for myself. I get this time alone when I exercise, especially when I run. At the end of January, although I could not run one mile without stopping, I signed up to run a half-marathon with Team in Training. I knew that the accountability of the training and fund-raising programs would force me to make time for running.

My tip for making exercise a priority is to put it on your schedule and make it part of your routine each week. During my half-marathon training, my husband and kids were still in bed when I would go for long runs early Saturday mornings. My proudest moment came after I crossed the finish line during that first half-marathon, and my daughter said she wanted to run a race, too, because she wanted to "win a medal like Mommy!"

My Healthy Tipping Point was when I realized that making healthy choices *now* will impact my kids for a lifetime. Teach your kids about nutrition *today* so they can make healthy choices when they start school or go off to college. Let your kids see you exercise *now*, and they will be more likely to exercise as teenagers and adults. Choose to be a healthy role model for your children so you can be there to watch them grow into healthy adults.

Healthy Shopping Lists

The first part of healthy eating is buying healthy foods; the second element is buying groceries in recipe-friendly combinations. People stare at a full fridge and complain there's nothing to eat because they didn't purchase food with a recipe-ready strategy in mind.

You've probably heard that grocery lists can shore up your impulse control, resulting in smaller grocery-bill tabs. In the same vein, a list can help you stick to healthier eating habits, since you're less likely to toss in that bag of cookies just "because it's on sale!" The key to really making shopping lists work for you is to couple them with meal planning. Now, meal planning sounds time-consuming, but it's actually only as complicated as you make it.

TOP FIVE RECIPES

Keep a list of the ingredients needed for your favorite recipes in your purse or wallet. You'll always know what you need to pick up at the store, even if you pop in without a list!

While some people choose to meal plan every breakfast, lunch, and dinner for the entire week, others meal plan in a more general way, determining flexible meal ideas in advance of a shopping trip. The concept behind general meal ideas is that many healthy options are actually quite similar on an ingredients level. So, at the very least, when you're making your healthy shopping lists, start by listing the ingredients for three or four meals you'd like to enjoy that week.

Once you've crafted your list, the next step is to compare it to the food you already have in your pantry. You might discover that you already do, in fact, have brown rice. Also, consider if there are any acceptable substitutions (for example, if a recipe called for zucchini and you've got a head of broccoli, swap it in).

Instead of relying on pricey frozen dinners, make a healthy casserole on Sunday and freeze individual servings to enjoy throughout the week.

The last step involves actually following your list at the store. A high percentage of list-users admit to buying "unexpected" purchases, not because they forgot to put the item on the list in the first place, but because they were tempted by displays and sales. Help ward off a spending free fall by building flexibility into your list. Allow yourself two fun foodie purchases, like an artisanal olive oil or a pint of ice cream, for example. List "two green vegetables" or "some type of berry" and select produce based on what's on sale and in season.

Provided below are two sample shopping lists: one for an individual and another for a family.

SAMPLE SHOPPING LIST NUMBER ONE
(FOR A ONE-PERSON HOUSEHOLD)

Meal Ideas:	Goat Cheese and Apricot Pizza (page 210) Perfect Baked Tofu (page 220) Sweet Potato and Black Bean Enchiladas (page 212) Millet veggie bowl (page 219)
Pantry	
Loaf of whole-grain bread	Whole-grain tortillas
Millet	Three cans of beans (pinto, chickpea, black)
Whole wheat flour	Salsa
Yeast	Spelt flour
Almonds	Jar of nut butter
Whole wheat pancake mix	Cashews
Dried apricots	Whole-grain cereal
Honey	Marinara sauce
Protein and Dairy	
Eggs	Four single-serving containers or one large container of Greek yogurt
Gallon of skim milk	Crumbled goat cheese
Hummus	Extra-firm tofu
Freezer	
Frozen strawberries	Frozen veggie patties
Frozen corn	
Produce	
Apples	Bananas
Berries (whatever is on sale)	Bagged raw spinach
Dark leafy greens (whatever is on sale)	Bagged arugula

Produce	
Sprouts	Two green vegetables (whatever is on sale)
Two sweet potatoes	Red and green peppers
Celery	Carrots
Pears	Tomatoes
Vidalia onion	
Fun Extras	
A bar of dark chocolate	Bottle of red wine

SAMPLE SHOPPING LIST NUMBER TWO
(FOR A HOUSEHOLD OF TWO ADULTS
AND ONE YOUNG CHILD)

Meal Ideas:	BBQ Tempeh Pizza (page 211) Couscous veggie bowl (page 218) No-Lettuce Double Bean Salad (page 206)
Pantry	
Two loaves whole-grain bread	Two packs of whole wheat tortillas
Couscous	Brown rice
Crackers	Six cans of beans (kidney, chickpea, black)
Whole wheat flour	Spelt flour
Yeast	Two jars of nut butter
Walnuts	Peanuts
Whole wheat pancake mix	Two boxes of whole-grain cereal
Raisins	Five cans of soup
Old-fashioned oatmeal	Marinara sauce
Whole wheat pasta	BBQ sauce
Protein and Dairy	
Eggs	Ten single-serving containers or three large containers of Greek yogurt
Gallon of skim milk	Swiss cheese
Shredded cheddar cheese	Two tubs of hummus

Protein and Dairy	
Two blocks of extra-firm tofu	Faux meat crumbles
Faux chicken tenders	Tempeh
Freezer	
Frozen strawberries	Frozen veggie patties
Frozen pineapple	Frozen corn
Frozen pizza	
Produce	
Apples	Bananas
Berries (whatever is on sale)	Bagged raw spinach
Zucchini	Squash
Dark leafy greens (whatever is on sale)	Five green vegetables (whatever is on sale)
Eggplant	Oranges
Avocados	Small red potatoes
Sweet potatoes	Carrots
Celery	Tomatoes
Pears	Cucumber
Red onion	Cilantro
Lime	
Fun Extras	
Gallon of coconut milk ice cream	Bag of all-natural potato chips

Healthy in the Kitchen

Fake, processed food is often called convenience food because it's, well, convenient. There's often little involved when you're serving up fake food. Real food, on the other hand, means prep work and cooking. Eating healthy, natural, real food does require you to spend some time in the kitchen. But don't run for the hills just yet!

Rest assured that cooking doesn't have to be time-consuming or difficult. Healthy meals can be fast and simple. Sure, there are complicated entrees that require hours in the kitchen, but there are many simple, wholesome meals that include less than five ingredients and go from fridge to plate in thirty minutes or less. There are many tools, appliances, and techniques that minimize prep work and cooking time. Don't forget that you can prepare a workweek's worth of dinners on Sunday and harvest the healthy rewards Monday through Friday!

Often, newbie cooks stay out of the kitchen simply because they feel confused by the process of cooking. I know that's why I avoided cooking for so many years! The fear of burning something or messing up a dish can be overwhelming. But guess what? No one is born knowing how to cook, and it is 100 percent possible to teach yourself how to make healthy, satisfying meals. The more you cook, the easier it will become. Don't be afraid of failing in the kitchen. Experimenting with new foods, tastes, and techniques is fun and exciting, if only you look at cooking in a positive light.

Worst-case scenario? You dump your burnt dinner in the trash and make a peanut butter and banana sandwich!

Cooking Techniques for the Newbie Cook

Baking/Roasting: Baking or roasting is a high-dry method of cooking in an oven. Generally, baking and roasting mean pretty much the same thing, but people use the term "baking" to refer to breads or cookies, and "roasting" to refer to vegetables or meat. The most important thing about baking or roasting is to remember to preheat the oven. It can take upward of ten minutes for an oven to reach the goal temperature, and if you put a food in too early, you can ruin the dish. And a reminder—the times listed below are just approximations; you should always follow a specific recipe's instructions for baking times and temperatures.

BAKING AND ROASTING TIMES

Food	Temperature and Length
Baked vegetables	375 to 400 degrees; 20–50 minutes
Baked potato	375 degrees; 50–75 minutes
Baked tofu	375 degrees; 20–35 minutes
Pizza	400 degrees; 15–20 minutes
Cookies	325 to 375 degrees; 7–15 minutes
Cake	350 degrees; 30–45 minutes

When baking vegetables, you'll want to give the veggies a light coating of canola or olive oil to ensure they don't dry out while cooking. Veggies are done when they start to turn golden brown. For baked goods, check the center with a toothpick or fork—if it comes out clean, it's cooked all the way.

BAKING TOFU

Tofu absorbs whatever flavors it is cooked with or marinated in, which makes it a versatile ingredient for plant eaters. For baking, you'll want to use extra-firm tofu. Unwrap and drain the tofu, and then place the block between several paper towels or clean cloths. Use heavy plates to press out the extra liquid. After 10–15 minutes, unwrap the tofu and cut into one-inch cubes. Let stand in a marinade, such as the one in Perfect Baked Tofu (page 220), Italian salad dressing, or BBQ sauce, for another ten minutes. Place on an oiled cookie sheet and bake at 375 for 30–40 minutes, until brown and crispy.

Alternatively, if you're short on time, you can skip the pressing method by slicing the tofu into very thin strips (quarter of an inch). Place the strips on an oiled cookie sheet and brush with a marinade. Bake at 375 degrees for 20–30 minutes, or until the edges look crunchy. This option is less flavorful but faster.

Only using half a block of tofu? Keep the remainder fresh by storing it in an airtight container filled with fresh water. Change the water daily. The tofu will keep fresh for up to a week.

Boiling: Boiling is the primary method for cooking grains, such as rice. You might also occasionally boil vegetables (although steaming is healthier because it locks in more nutrients), especially potatoes for mashed pota-toes. When boiling, make sure the pot is large enough to fit all the food plus enough water to cover the food completely. The water shouldn't reach the top of the pot—it will boil over. Covering the pot with a lid will make the water boil faster. Always wait until the water is boiling to add the food.

Steaming: Steaming is a very fast and healthy way to cook vegetables. To steam, fill a wok or pot with a half to one cup of water—just enough to line the bottom. Cover with a lid and bring to a boil. Then, add the chopped vegetables to the pot, re-cover, and cook for five to ten minutes. When you can easily push a fork into the vegetable, it's ready. Scoop out the vegetables or carefully drain in a colander.

STEAMED DARK LEAFY GREENS

Kale, collard greens, and Swiss chard are delicious . . . if they are cooked correctly—otherwise, they taste like mush! Thoroughly rinse and chop the greens. Then, fill a pot with a quarter cup of water, bring to a boil, add greens, and cover with a lid. After ten minutes, remove from the heat and drain. Salt the greens or add a dash of soy sauce.

Stir-Frying: When you stir-fry, you cook on the stove-top at high heat with a small amount of oil. Stir-frying can be done in a skillet or a wok. Don't go overboard with the olive or canola oil—add just a tablespoon. You'll want to stir the food constantly to prevent it from sticking to the pan bottom.

You can also make scrambled eggs using a stir-fry method. Simply crack eggs into an oiled, hot wok or griddle and use a wooden spoon to blend and stir. Right before the eggs firm up, add a dash of milk or milk substitute and stir thoroughly.

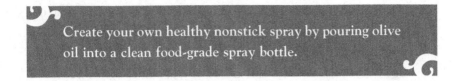

Create your own healthy nonstick spray by pouring olive oil into a clean food-grade spray bottle.

Healthy Cooking Swaps and Easy Shortcuts

- **Cook Ahead:** The easiest way to eat healthy? Bake extras! Next time you're preparing dinner, make a double batch of the entire meal and have leftovers for lunch. You can also freeze extra servings in airtight containers and eat weeks down the road. Many busy workers or parents find it helpful to cook on a Sunday night and freeze meals for the rest of the week. You can even freeze cooked grains!

- **Read the Recipe:** Read the recipe's ingredients list and directions at least twice. To make sure you're not missing a key item, set out all the ingredients before you begin. Always begin with the food that will take the longest to prepare, such as the rice; this way, you can prepare the other foods while the rice is simmering away.

- **Fake Frying:** Breaded, fried foods are delicious, but they're not very healthy. To fake the taste and texture of a fried food, dip the food (such as tofu or a meat or vegetable) in beaten egg whites and then coat with panko crumbs. If you're using bread crumbs, be sure to check the ingredients for trans fat. Place the breaded food on an oiled cookie sheet and bake at 375 degrees for 30–45 minutes.

- **Know When to Be Exact:** When baking bread or cookies, it's important to measure out every ingredient exactly as the recipe calls for. For dishes like pastas, soups, and stir-fries, it's not necessary to be so precise. Don't waste time measuring ingredients perfectly for such dishes; you can eyeball it (a tablespoon looks like half a golf ball and a cup looks like a baseball).

- **Applesauce Instead of Oil:** When baking cake or cookies, swap out the oil for equal parts of applesauce. It only mildly impacts the flavor and texture.
- **Egg Substitutions:** To create a "vegan egg," simply mix three table-spoons of ground flaxseed with one tablespoon of water. Let the mixture stand until a gel forms, and then add to bread, cookie, pan-cakes, waffles, or cake recipes as you normally would. Alternatively, one-quarter cup of mashed ripe banana often works well as an egg substitute.
- **Milk Substitutions:** You can sub out cow's milk for equal parts soy, almond, coconut, hemp, or other milk substitutes.
- **Hummus Instead of Cheese:** In casseroles and pastas, swap out the cheese for equal parts hummus, especially white bean varieties. Hummus creates a creamy, rich texture and even mimics Alfredo sauce!

Scout online classified ads or garage sales to score high-quality appliances at a discount.

Eight

HEALTHY RECIPES AND MEAL IDEAS

Healthy and Hearty Breakfasts

Breakfast is oh so important to your healthy journey—don't skip it! People who eat breakfast are, on average, a healthier weight than people who don't; additionally, breakfast eaters actually live longer. Eating a healthy and hearty breakfast will stabilize your blood sugar, which enables you to easily make healthier choices all day long.

On days you're pressed for time, try one of these very simple—but healthy—breakfasts:

- Two slices of whole wheat toast with peanut butter and fresh fruit;
- Whole-grain cereal with two tablespoons chopped almonds, sliced banana or strawberries, and milk or milk substitute;
- Greek yogurt (higher in protein than regular) with raw oatmeal (the yogurt will soften it) or whole-grain cereal and fruit;
- A smoothie; for recipes, check out pages 232–36.

Please don't relegate the following hot breakfast recipes to the weekend! True, some require twenty minutes of baking time, but these meals demand only a few minutes of prep work. So, pull your meal together, pop it in the oven, and jump in the shower. When you're done, your meal will be, too. And there's nothing better on a Monday morning than a delicious, hot breakfast.

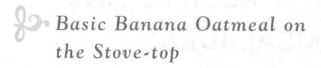

Basic Banana Oatmeal on the Stove-top

For 1 serving (per serving: 300 calories; 4 g fat; 10 g protein; 60 g carbohydrates; 7 g fiber)

½ cup old-fashioned oatmeal
½ cup water
½ cup milk or milk substitute
1 ripe banana, thinly sliced

DIRECTIONS

In a small saucepan, combine all the ingredients and stir together. Over a medium heat and stirring occasionally, simmer until the liquid is absorbed (about five minutes).

Mix It Up: *Healthy topping options for oatmeal are almost endless. Try a scoop of peanut butter, unsweetened coconut, flaxseed or chia seeds (which provide heart-healthy omega-3s), fresh berries, nuts, a few chocolate chips, a sprinkle of cinnamon, a drizzle of maple syrup, or a tablespoon of crunchy granola.*

Basic Banana Oatmeal in the Microwave

For 1 serving (per serving: 280 calories; 4 g fat; 8 g protein; 58 g carbohydrates; 7 g fiber)

½ cup old-fashioned oatmeal
¼ cup water
¼ cup milk or milk substitute
1 ripe banana, thinly sliced

DIRECTIONS

In a glass microwave-safe bowl, combine the oatmeal, water, and milk. Stir.

Microwave for 2–2½ minutes, remove from microwave, and stir again.

Thinly slice the banana and stir it into the oatmeal. Let stand one minute before serving.

Mexican Breakfast Burrito

For 1 serving (per serving: 385 calories; 17 g fat; 21 g protein; 40 g carbohydrates; 9 g fiber)

¼ tablespoon olive or canola oil
¼ cup thinly sliced red pepper
¼ cup thinly sliced green pepper
½ cup chopped portabella mushrooms
2 eggs

¼ cup canned black beans, drained and rinsed

2 tablespoons jarred salsa

1 whole wheat wrap

DIRECTIONS

Preheat the stove-top to medium high.

In a frying pan over medium-high heat combine the oil and the red and green peppers. Cook for 3 minutes. Add the mushrooms and cook for another 5 minutes, stirring occasionally.

In a small bowl, lightly whisk the eggs. Add the eggs to the vegetable mix and scramble until the eggs set.

In the center of a whole wheat wrap, combine the eggs and vegetable mix with the black beans. Top with salsa and roll up the wrap.

Homemade Almond Butter Granola

For 10 half-cup servings (per serving: 250 calories; 15 g fat; 7 g of protein; 26 g of carbohydrates; 4 g of fiber)

½ cup almond butter

¼ cup maple syrup

1 teaspoon cinnamon

¾ teaspoon salt (if almond butter is salted, skip or reduce the salt)

3 cups old-fashioned oatmeal

1 cup slivered almonds

DIRECTIONS

Preheat the oven to 300 degrees.

In a small saucepan over a low heat, combine the almond butter, maple syrup, cinnamon, and salt. Stir thoroughly until melted and well combined.

Pour in the oatmeal and stir until thoroughly mixed.

Spread the mixture evenly on an oiled cookie sheet and bake for 35 minutes, stirring occasionally to keep it from burning.

Turn off the oven. Remove the cookie sheet from the oven and sprinkle the almonds on top. Return the cookie sheet to the oven and let the mix rest for an hour. Once the granola has cooled completely, store it in airtight container. It will keep for four days.

> **Mix It Up:** *This granola tastes fabulous with vanilla Greek yogurt or ice-cold almond milk. For variety, use different types of nut butter, like peanut butter or sunflower butter.*

Toasted Quinoa and Pumpkin Yogurt

For 1 serving (per serving: 460 calories; 14 g fat; 23 g protein; 64 g carbohydrates; 6 g of fiber)

¼ cup uncooked quinoa
1 tablespoon maple syrup
¼ cup canned pumpkin puree, chilled
One 6-ounce serving vanilla yogurt (Greek, if possible)
¼ tablespoon cinnamon
2 tablespoons chopped pecans

DIRECTIONS
Preheat the oven to 375 degrees.

Rinse the quinoa if it's not prerinsed. In a small bowl, combine the quinoa and maple syrup. Spread the mix out evenly on the bottom of an oiled glass casserole dish and bake for 15 minutes.

Meanwhile, in a small bowl, combine the pumpkin puree, yogurt, and cinnamon.

Remove the casserole dish from oven and let it cool for 15 minutes.

Top the toasted quinoa with the pumpkin yogurt and serve in a bowl with a sprinkle of pecans.

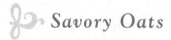 Savory Oats

For 1 serving (per serving: 270 calories; 11 g fat; 20 g protein; 32 g carbohydrates; 5 g fiber)

   ½ cup old-fashioned oatmeal
   ½ cup water
   ¼ cup 1 percent fat cottage cheese
   ¼ cup raw spinach, torn into smaller pieces
   Pinch of pepper
   1 egg
   1 tablespoon milk or milk substitute
   1 green scallion, chopped

DIRECTIONS

In a small saucepan, combine the oatmeal, water, cottage cheese, spinach, and pepper. Stir, and turn heat to medium.

Stirring occasionally, cook the oat mixture until all the liquid is absorbed (about 5 minutes).

As the oats are cooking, beat the egg and the milk in a small bowl. Pour the mixture into a medium-hot oiled frying pan, and scramble.

Scoop the oatmeal into a serving bowl and top with the eggs and scallions.

Mix It Up: *Top with hot sauce or salsa for spicy oats.*

Green and Red Quiche Cornbread

For 4 servings (per serving: 400 calories; 20 g fat; 21 g protein; 60 g carbohydrates; 5 g fiber)

   2 cups dry cornbread mix
   2 cups raw spinach, torn into smaller pieces
   1 small tomato, chopped
   4 eggs, beaten
   ¼ cup milk or milk substitute
   ½ cup shredded cheddar cheese
   Salt and pepper to taste

DIRECTIONS

Preheat the oven to 350 degrees.

Prepare the cornbread mix according to package directions. Then, pour evenly into an oiled cast-iron skillet and bake for 15 minutes.

In a small bowl, combine the spinach, tomato, beaten eggs, milk, cheese, salt, and pepper.

Pour the egg mix on top of the cornbread.

Return the quiche cornbread to the oven and bake for 20 minutes.

Remove the skillet from the oven and let the dish stand for 5 minutes before slicing into quarters and serving.

Sweet Potato Pancake

For 1 serving (per serving: 520 calories; 21 g fat; 17 g protein; 71 g carbohydrates; 10 g fiber)

- ¾ cup old-fashioned oats
- 2 tablespoons milk or milk substitute
- ¼ cup sweet potato, cooked and mashed (To cook a sweet potato quickly, wash the potato, prick it with a fork several times, wrap it in paper towel, and microwave on medium for approximately 6 minutes, or until it's softened enough to mash.)
- 2 tablespoons pecans, crushed
- 1 egg
- ¼ tablespoon cinnamon
- Four strawberries, sliced
- 1 tablespoon maple syrup

DIRECTIONS

Oil a frying pan and turn the heat to medium high.

In a medium bowl, mix the oats, milk, mashed sweet potato, pecans, egg, and cinnamon.

Scoop the mix into the pan and use a heat-resistant spatula to form a pancake.

Adjust the heat to medium and cook the pancake for approximately 10 minutes, or until the bottom begins to brown (use a spatula to gently lift up the edges of the pancake to check).

Flip the pancake by turning the frying pan over a plate. If need be, use the spatula to gently ease the pancake onto the plate. Return the pancake to the pan and cook the other side for several more minutes, until golden brown.

Top the pancake with the strawberries and maple syrup.

Peanut Butter French Toast

For 1 serving (per serving: 490 calories; 18 g fat; 26 g protein; 57 g carbohydrates; 7 g fiber)

- 1 tablespoon peanut butter
- 1 egg
- 1 tablespoon milk or milk substitute
- 2 slices whole wheat bread
- 3 ounces vanilla yogurt (preferably Greek)

DIRECTIONS

Oil a frying pan and place it over medium-high heat.

In a medium microwavable bowl, heat the peanut butter for 30 seconds on medium, until creamy. Add the egg and milk and whisk.

Dip each slice of bread into the peanut butter mixture, coating both sides as thoroughly as possible.

Place the bread slices in the frying pan. Evenly spread any remaining peanut butter mixture on top of the bread slices.

Cook for 3–4 minutes per side, until golden brown.

Top with yogurt.

No-Egg French Toast

For 1 serving (per serving: 510 calories; 6 g fat; 10 g protein; 110 g carbohydrates; 8 g fiber)

   1 overly ripe banana
   2 tablespoons milk or milk substitute
   ¼ tablespoon cinnamon
   ½ tablespoon honey
   2 slices whole wheat bread
   2 tablespoons maple syrup

DIRECTIONS

Generously oil a frying pan and place it over medium-high heat.

In a food processor or blender, combine the banana, milk, cinnamon, and honey and pulse until a thick liquid forms.

Dip each slice of bread into the banana mixture, coating both sides as thoroughly as possible.

Place the bread in the frying pan. Spread any remaining banana mixture evenly on the top of each bread slice.

Cook for 3–4 minutes per side, until golden brown. The bread may be difficult to flip because it tends to stick to the pan—be careful!

Serve with maple syrup.

Goat Cheese Frittata

For 4 servings (per serving: 235 calories; 17 g of fat; 17 g of protein; 3 g of carbohydrates; 1 g of fiber)

> 1 tablespoon olive or canola oil
> 2 cups zucchini, thinly sliced into rounds
> 8 eggs
> ¼ cup chopped scallions
> ½ cup crumbled goat cheese
> ½ teaspoon salt
> ¼ tablespoon fresh ground pepper

DIRECTIONS

Preheat the oven to a high broil.

Pour the oil into a 12-inch cast-iron skillet on the stove-top, and turn the heat to medium high. Add the zucchini slices and cook for 5 minutes, stirring occasionally.

In a large bowl, lightly whisk the eggs. Add the scallions, goat cheese, salt, and pepper, and stir thoroughly.

Pour the egg mixture over the zucchini slices. Do not stir! Cook at medium high for approximately 10 minutes, or until the egg mixture is set throughout.

Place the cast-iron skillet in the oven and broil for 3–5 minutes, or until the top is browned. Carefully remove the pan from the oven and let it stand for several minutes before serving.

Mix It Up: *Swap the goat cheese for another type of shredded cheese— white, cheddar, or a Mexican cheese blend. You can also swap in other vegetables, such as red pepper, broccoli, spinach, or squash.*

Refreshing Salads

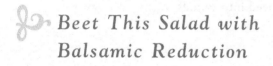 *Beet This Salad with Balsamic Reduction*

For 1 serving (per serving, without the dressing: 435 calories; 23 g fat; 20 g protein; 42 g carbohydrates; 14 g fiber)

SALAD
4 medium beets
2 cups packed raw baby spinach
1 carrot, thinly sliced
¼ cup crumbled goat cheese
2 tablespoons chopped pecans

DRESSING
2 tablespoons Balsamic Reduction (see recipe on page 224).

DIRECTIONS
Scrub the beets, place them in a large saucepan, and fill with water to just cover beets. Bring to a boil. Boil for no more than 15–20 minutes; do not

overcook. Once a fork can be inserted, the beets are done. Drain and let the beets cool. Remove the skins by rubbing the beets with a paper towel and then slice them into quarters.

Combine the spinach, beets, carrot, goat cheese, and pecans on a plate.

Drizzle with 2 tablespoons of Balsamic Reduction.

Strawberry Fields Salad with Citrus Poppy Seed Dressing

For 1 serving (per serving, without dressing: 250 calories; 13 g fat; 10 g protein; 28 g carbohydrates; 10 g fiber)

SALAD
¼ cup sliced almonds
1 cup packed romaine lettuce, torn into small pieces
1 cup arugula
5 strawberries, greens removed and sliced
2 stalks celery, chopped
¼ cup canned chickpeas, rinsed and drained

DRESSING
2 tablespoons Citrus Poppy Seed Dressing (see recipe on page 223).

DIRECTIONS
Turn the oven to a low broil. Place the almonds on a cookie sheet and broil for 2–3 minutes. Do not overcook!

Combine the romaine lettuce, arugula, strawberries, celery, almonds, and chickpeas on a plate.

Drizzle with 2 tablespoons of dressing and serve.

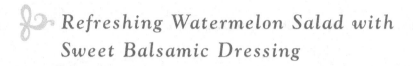 ## Refreshing Watermelon Salad with Sweet Balsamic Dressing

For 1 serving (per serving without dressing: 165 calories; 9 g fat; 8 g protein; 15 g carbohydrates; 3 g fiber)

SALAD
2 cups packed raw baby spinach
¼ cup packed fresh basil, chopped
1 cup cubed watermelon
¼ cup feta cheese

DRESSING
2 tablespoons Sweet Balsamic Dressing (see recipe on page 223).

DIRECTIONS
Combine the spinach, basil, watermelon, and feta on a plate.

Drizzle with 2 tablespoons of dressing and serve.

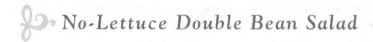 ## No-Lettuce Double Bean Salad

For 1 serving (per serving: 300 calories; 15 g fat; 10 g protein; 34 g carbohydrates; 10 g fiber)

¼ cup frozen corn
¼ cup canned black beans, drained and rinsed

¼ cup canned kidney beans, drained and rinsed

½ medium tomato, seeded and chopped

½ cup peeled and chopped cucumber

2 tablespoons chopped red onion

1 tablespoon chopped fresh cilantro

1 tablespoon olive or canola oil

Juice of 1 lime

Dash of pepper

DIRECTIONS

Defrost the frozen corn by putting it in a colander set up in the sink. Let warm water run through the kernels until they are soft.

In a medium bowl, combine the corn, black and kidney beans, tomato, cucumber, onion, cilantro, oil, lime juice, and pepper. Stir thoroughly to distribute the flavors evenly.

Plate the salad and serve.

Warm Roasted Vegetable Salad with Caramelized Pecans

For 1 serving (per serving: 535 calories; 31 g fat; 10 g protein; 60 g carbohydrates; 13 g fiber)

1 small sweet potato, unpeeled and cubed into bite-size pieces

2 carrots, peeled and chopped

1 cup chopped broccoli

1 tablespoon olive or canola oil

2 tablespoons chopped pecans

½ tablespoon butter or butter substitute

1 tablespoon sugar
Pinch of salt
¼ cup apple juice
¼ cup cannellini beans, drained and rinsed

DIRECTIONS
Preheat the oven to 375 degrees.

In a medium bowl, combine the chopped sweet potato, carrots, and broccoli. Toss with oil.

Spoon the vegetable mix evenly onto an oiled cookie sheet and place in
the oven. Cook for 25 minutes.

As the vegetables are roasting, caramelize the pecans. In a small saucepan,
cook the pecans, butter, sugar, and salt on medium low. Stir constantly until
the sugar dissolves completely, about 3–5 minutes. Transfer the nuts to a
plate and allow to cool.

Heat the apple juice on the stove-top on medium heat or in the microwave.

When the vegetables are done, scoop them into a large bowl, mix in the
beans, and add the heated apple juice. Stir thoroughly to combine.

Plate and top with the caramelized pecans.

Hot Meals

½ and ½ Pizza Dough (with Cheese Pizza variation)

For 6 personal pizzas (per serving: 320 calories; 4 g fat; 5 g protein; 65 g carbohydrates; 6 g fiber)

FOR PIZZA DOUGH
1 package of active dry yeast
¼ cup plus 1½ cups warm
  (not hot) water
1 tablespoon honey
1 tablespoon vegetable oil
½ tablespoon salt
2 cups organic all-purpose
  white flour
2 cups spelt flour

FOR CHEESE PIZZA
1½ cups store-bought
  marinara
1½ cups shredded cheese
  (cheddar, mozzarella, or
  other variety)

DIRECTIONS FOR THE DOUGH
Preheat the oven to 400 degrees.

In a small bowl, combine the packet of dry yeast with the ¼ cup warm water and honey. Give the mixture a good stir and let it stand for exactly 10 minutes.

When the yeast is nearly ready, combine 1½ cups warm water and the vegetable oil, salt, and flours in the mixer bowl of a stand mixer with the hook attachment. (Alternatively, you can use a wooden spoon to mix the dough; mix with an upward-thrusting motion.)

Add the yeast to the flour mix and stir for 2 minutes, until a sticky and stiff dough forms.

Separate the dough into six balls and place them in an oiled glass casserole dish. Cover the dish with a clean towel and place it in a warm spot (on top of the dryer or the heater or in a prewarmed oven turned off). Let the dough rise for an hour before preparing the pizzas. Unbaked dough can be placed in tightly sealed plastic bags and frozen for several months.

DIRECTIONS FOR THE CHEESE PIZZAS
Preheat oven to 400 degrees.

Roll out each dough ball to form a flat, thin circle. Place each on an oiled cookie sheet or a pizza stone.

Top each pizza with ¼ cup marinara sauce and ¼ cup cheese, bake for 15 minutes, and serve.

> **Mix It Up:** *Think beyond the flat pizza—trying creating calzones, which freeze well after baking. Calzones are pizza pockets stuffed with sauce, cheese, and veggies. To make a calzone, prepare the pizza dough following the instructions above and separate into six small balls of dough. Roll out each ball and scoop the stuffing ingredients (sauce, cheese, and toppings) onto one half of the circle. Fold over the other half, press the stuffed dough pocket closed, and use a fork to seal the edges. Bake on an oiled cookie sheet at 400 degrees for 20 minutes, or until the calzone browns.*

 Goat Cheese and Apricot Pizza

For 1 personal pizza (per serving: 500 calories; 12 g fat; 12 g protein; 88 g carbohydrates; 8 g fiber)

⅙ of the ½ and ½ Pizza Dough recipe (see page 209)
½ tablespoon honey

¼ cup store-bought marinara sauce

4 dried apricot halves, chopped fine

¼ cup packed arugula

1 ounce crumbled goat cheese

DIRECTIONS

Preheat the oven to 400 degrees.

On a lightly floured surface, roll out the pizza dough to form a thin circle. Transfer to a lightly oiled cookie sheet or pizza stone.

In a small bowl, combine the honey and the marinara sauce. Spread the mixture evenly on the pizza dough.

Top the pizza with the apricots, arugula, and goat cheese.

Bake for 17 minutes.

BBQ Tempeh Pizza

For 1 personal pizza (per serving: 600 calories; 22 g fat; 24 g protein; 79 g carbohydrates; 8 g fiber)

⅙ of ½ and ½ Pizza Dough recipe (see page 209)

2 tablespoons store-bought BBQ sauce

1 tablespoon store-bought marinara sauce

¼ (8-ounce) package tempeh, crumbled

2 tablespoons frozen corn

¼ cup cheddar cheese

DIRECTIONS

Preheat the oven to 400 degrees.

On a lightly floured surface, roll out the pizza dough to form a thin circle. Transfer to a lightly oiled cookie sheet or pizza stone.

In a small bowl, combine 1 tablespoon each of the BBQ sauce and the marinara sauce. Spread evenly on the pizza dough.

In another small bowl, combine the tempeh and 1 tablespoon of the BBQ sauce. Spoon evenly on top of the pizza sauce.

Top the pizza with the frozen corn and cheddar cheese.

Bake for 17 minutes.

Sweet Potato and Black Bean Enchiladas

For 4 servings (per serving: 375 calories; 4 g fat; 15 g protein; 75 g carbohydrates; 16 g fiber)

ENCHILADAS
2 large sweet potatoes, skinned and cubed
1 can black beans, drained and rinsed
½ cup frozen corn
½ cup chopped Vidalia onion
4 large whole wheat tortillas

Smooth Salsa

4 large tomatoes, chopped

2 tablespoons chopped Vidalia onion

2 tablespoons canned green chiles

¼ cup packed cilantro

2 tablespoons fresh lime juice

½ tablespoon salt

DIRECTIONS

Preheat oven to 375 degrees.

Bring a medium saucepan of water to a boil and add the sweet potato cubes. Boil the sweet potatoes for 15 minutes, or until they are soft.

In a medium bowl, mash together the sweet potatoes, black beans, frozen corn, and onion.

Oil a glass casserole dish.

Scoop ¼ of the potato mixture into the center of a tortilla and roll it up. Place the tortilla in the casserole dish, with edge of tortilla down so it stays in a roll. Repeat to make the other tortillas, and pack the tortillas tightly in the casserole dish to keep the ends from unraveling.

To prepare the Smooth Salsa, combine all the salsa ingredients in a blender or food processor and pulse until the ingredients are finely blended. Pour the salsa evenly over the tortillas.

Bake for 15 minutes. Serve warm.

℘ Southwestern Casserole

For 6 servings (per serving: 300 calories; 14 g fat; 16 g protein; 30 g carbohydrates;
6 g fiber)

½ cup coarsely chopped red onion
1 tablespoon minced garlic
½ tablespoon olive or canola oil
½ tablespoon chili powder
½ tablespoon pepper
½ tablespoon salt
½ can (8 ounces) red kidney beans, drained and rinsed
½ can (8 ounces) black beans, drained and rinsed
½ cup thawed frozen corn
1½ cups brown rice, cooked
¾ cup milk or milk substitute
2 eggs, beaten
1½ cups shredded cheddar cheese
½ cup coarsely chopped green pepper

DIRECTIONS
Preheat the oven to 350 degrees.

In a frying pan on high heat, combine the onion, garlic, and oil. Cook until
the onion browns, about 3 minutes.

In a large bowl, combine the onion mixture, seasonings, beans, corn, cooked
brown rice, milk, eggs, cheese, and green pepper.

Pour the mixture into an oiled large glass casserole dish.

Bake for 45 minutes, or until the top begins to brown. Serve warm.

Veggie Bowls

Make large batches of grains, like rice, ahead of time and freeze leftovers in an airtight container for up to three months. Reheat by warming in a skillet with a dash of water.

A veggie bowl is one of the healthiest meals around because you can pack it with a little bit of all things nutritious—whole grains, protein, dairy, veggies, and nuts. This wholesome meal is also very convenient. You can make a big batch, store it in the fridge for up to five days, and enjoy veggie bowls for lunches or dinners throughout the week. No matter what's in it, a veggie bowl tastes great warmed or chilled.

Veggie bowls don't even have to be served in a bowl! Try these tasty variations:

- **Veggie Bowl Salad:** Serve the chilled mixture over spinach or another type of salad green.
- **Veggie Bowl Burrito:** Roll up the warmed mixture in a whole wheat or corn tortilla.
- **Veggie Bowl Casserole:** For two servings, combine 2½ cups of prepared veggie bowl mixture with two eggs, ¾ cup milk, and 1½ cups shredded cheese. Bake in a small baking dish at 350 degrees for 25–35 minutes, or until the casserole top browns.

You can customize veggie bowls to suit your tastes and diet. From the following chart, choose one base, one protein, one nut, one dairy, as many veggies as you wish, and a salsa or sauce. You'll find recipes following the chart. There are many other options for veggie bowl mix-ins—the only limit is your culinary imagination!

Here are some stand-out veggie bowl ideas:

- Millet, chickpeas, almonds, grilled zucchini and yellow squash, Green Secret Sauce (page 223; served chilled);
- Quinoa, Carolina BBQ Baked Tofu (page 221), blue cheese, carrots, tomatoes, grilled pineapple, Carolina BBQ Sauce (page 224; served warm);
- Brown rice, black beans, cheddar cheese, raw red and green peppers, raw onions, boiled corn, Pico de Gallo (page 222; served warm);
- Couscous, boiled egg, sunflower seeds, goat cheese, spinach, carrots, raisins, red onion, and Sweet Balsamic Dressing (page 223; served chilled)

MAKE YOUR OWN VEGGIE BOWL

REFER TO PAGES 220–24 FOR RECIPES FOR ITEMS IN ITALICS.

BASE (Select 1)		
Barley	Couscous	Quinoa
Brown rice	Lentils	Wheat berries
Buckwheat	Millet	Wild rice
PROTEIN (Select 1)		
Azuki beans	Scrambled egg	Navy beans
Perfect Baked Tofu	Kidney beans	*Carolina BBQ Baked Tofu*
Chickpeas	Black beans	Boiled egg
Sweet Tempeh		

NUTS		
(Optional or Select 1)		
Sunflower seeds	Walnuts	Peanuts
Almonds	Pecans	Pine nuts
Cashews		

DAIRY		
(Optional or Select 1)		
Blue cheese	Dollop of plain yogurt or sour cream	Buffalo mozzarella
Feta cheese		Goat cheese
Cheddar cheese		

VEGGIES AND FRUITS	
(Select Many)	
Green peas (steamed)	Spinach (raw or steamed)
Red, green, yellow peppers (raw, grilled, or baked)	Tomatoes (raw or sun-dried)
Eggplant (baked or stir-fried)	Squash and zucchini (raw or stir-fried)
Kale (raw and rubbed with sea salt and olive oil or steamed)	Avocado (raw)
Sprouts (raw)	Berries (raw)
Sweet or white potatoes (baked)	Sliced apples (raw)
Carrots (raw, grilled, or baked)	Peaches (raw or grilled)
Corn (fresh or boiled)	Raisins or other dried fruit
	Pineapple (raw or grilled)
	Corn (raw or boiled)

SALSAS AND SAUCES		
(Select 1)		
Carolina BBQ Sauce	Jarred store-bought pasta sauce	Bottled BBQ sauce
Pico de Gallo		*Citrus Poppy Seed Dressing*
Bottled salad dressing	*Balsamic Reduction*	
Sweet Balsamic Dressing	*Green Secret Sauce*	

GLUTEN FREE

Brown rice, wild rice, quinoa, millet, and buckwheat are naturally gluten free; instructions on how to prepare these grains are provided below. Other gluten-free grains include amaranth, sorghum, and teff.

COOKING INSTRUCTIONS FOR VEGGIE BOWL BASES

Base Type	Preparation for One Serving
Barley: A nutritious whole grain, barley is very chewy and flavorful. It's traditionally used in soups and stews, but tastes great in a veggie bowl, too.	In a medium saucepan, bring ¾ cup of water to a boil; add ¼ cup barley (measured dry); cover tightly and turn down the heat to medium-low; simmer for 30–40 minutes, until the barley is soft and the water evaporates. Fluff with a fork and serve.
Brown rice: Chewier and nuttier-tasting than white rice, brown rice is a whole, natural grain.	Same as for barley, above.
Buckwheat: Despite its name, buckwheat isn't actually wheat at all—it's a seed of a plant in the herb family. Buckwheat has a very distinct flavor and soft texture.	In a medium saucepan, bring ¾ cup water to a boil and add ¼ cup buckwheat (measured dry); cover tightly and turn down heat to medium-low; simmer for 15 minutes. Remove from the heat and let stand covered for another 10 minutes. Drain away any excess liquid, fluff with a fork, and serve.
Couscous: Although couscous may look like a grain, it's semolina from durum wheat, the primary ingredient in pasta.	In a medium saucepan, bring ⅓ cup water to a boil. Remove from the heat, add ¼ cup couscous (measured dry), and cover tightly. Let stand for 5 minutes, fluff with a fork, and serve.
Lentils: Technically a legume, lentils come in green, brown, red, and yellow varieties. As lentils cook, they absorb liquid flavors readily. So for extra flavor, try adding spices like curry to the water, or swapping in vegetable broth for water.	In a medium saucepan, combine ¼ cup lentils with ⅓ cup water and bring to a boil. Cover and simmer for 25 minutes, or until the lentils are soft and the water has been absorbed.

Base Type	Preparation for Two Servings
Millet: Millet is high in protein and vitamin B. Millet fluffs up like rice when cooked, but be careful not to overcook it, because millet quickly becomes mushy.	In a medium saucepan, bring 1 cup water to a rolling boil and add ¼ cup millet (measured dry). Boil for 20 minutes, drain the excess water, and return to the stove-top. Turn off the heat and allow the excess water to evaporate. Fluff with a fork and serve.
Quinoa: Technically a seed, quinoa (pronounced "KEEN-*wah*") has a slightly nutty flavor and a fluffy texture.	To keep the birds and pests away, quinoa seeds have a soapy coating. You might need to rinse quinoa prior to cooking by swishing it around in cold water and draining. To cook: In a medium saucepan, bring 1 cup water to a rolling boil and add in ¼ cup quinoa (measured dry). Boil for 10 minutes, drain excess water, and return to the stove-top. Turn off the heat and allow the excess water to evaporate. Fluff with a fork and serve.
Wheat berries: Wheat berries are whole wheat kernels that look like thick pieces of brown rice. They are extremely chewy and taste great cold or warm.	In a medium saucepan, bring 2 cups water to a boil. Add ¼ cup wheat berries (measured dry) and boil for 1 hour. Drain any excess liquid, fluff with a fork, and serve.
Wild rice: Similar to brown rice in texture, wild rice is chewier, more flavorful, and more nutrient-dense than white rice. Did you know that wild rice is actually a grass?	Same as brown rice, although wild rice may take longer to cook.

RECIPES FOR VEGGIE BOWL PROTEINS

Protein	Preparation for One Serving
Perfect Baked Tofu	*Per serving: 315 calories; 15 g fat; 14 g protein; 37 g carbohydrates; 1 g fiber* ⅓ (15-ounce) block extra-firm tofu ½ tablespoon olive oil 2 tablespoons honey ½ tablespoon chili powder ¼ tablespoon black pepper 1 tablespoon sesame seeds DIRECTIONS Preheat the oven to 375 degrees and oil a cookie sheet. Remove the tofu from its packaging. Wrap it in several paper towels and place between two heavy plates to press away extra liquid. Let stand at least 10 minutes. To make the marinade: In a medium bowl, combine the oil, honey, chili powder, and pepper. Slice the tofu into 1-inch cubes and add to the marinade bowl, coating the cubes completely. Place the tofu cubes on the cookie sheet and sprinkle with the sesame seeds. Bake for 30–40 minutes or until the tofu is brown and crispy.

Protein	Preparation for One Serving
Carolina BBQ Baked Tofu	*Per serving: 210 calories; 9 g fat; 15 g protein; 21 g carbohydrates; 2 g fiber*

⅓ (15-ounce) block extra-firm tofu
2 tablespoons yellow mustard
½ tablespoon molasses
½ tablespoon honey
½ tablespoon cider vinegar
1 teaspoon chili powder
½ teaspoon cayenne pepper
Heavy pinches of dried oregano, salt, and pepper

DIRECTIONS
Preheat the oven to 375 degrees and oil a cookie sheet.

Remove the tofu from its packaging. Wrap it in several paper towels and place between two heavy plates to press away extra liquid. Let stand at least 10 minutes.

To make the marinade: In a medium bowl, combine the mustard, molasses, honey, vinegar, and seasonings.

Slice the tofu into 1-inch cubes and add to the marinade bowl, coating the cubes completely. Place the tofu cubes on the cookie sheet.

Bake for 30–40 minutes or until the tofu is brown and crispy.

Protein	Preparation for One Serving
Sweet Tempeh	*Per serving: 320 calories; 18 g fat; 19 g protein; 28 g carbohydrates; 1 g fiber* ½ (8-ounce) package tempeh 1 tablespoon maple syrup ¼ cup lemon juice ½ tablespoon olive oil ½ tablespoon chopped fresh rosemary Pinch salt and pepper DIRECTIONS Slice the tempeh lengthwise to create two thick pieces. Then cut into ½-inch strips. In a medium bowl, combine the remaining ingredients to make the marinade. Add the tempeh to the marinade bowl and coat thoroughly. Let the tempeh stand for 15 minutes. Heat a wok to medium high and oil it. Add the tempeh and marinade and cook for 8–10 minutes, flipping halfway through, until the tempeh begins to brown and the marinade has been absorbed.

RECIPES FOR VEGGIE BOWL SALSAS AND SAUCES

Salsas and Sauces	Preparation
Pico de Gallo	*For eight 2-tablespoon servings (per serving: 15 calories; 1 g fat; 1 g protein; 2 g carbohydrates; 0.5 g fiber)* 1 large tomato, seeded and diced ¼ cup diced red onion ½ tablespoon chopped fresh jalapeño pepper 1 tablespoon finely chopped fresh cilantro 2 tablespoons lime juice ½ tablespoon olive oil Dash salt and pepper DIRECTIONS Combine all the ingredients in a small bowl. Cover and refrigerate for at least an hour, stirring several times to create a rich flavor and texture.

Salsas and Sauces	Preparation
Citrus Poppy Seed Dressing	*For six 2-tablespoon servings (per serving: 115 calories; 10 g fat; 0.5 g protein; 7 g carbohydrates; 0.2 g fiber)* 2 tablespoons white sugar ½ cup orange juice 1 tablespoon chopped white onion ½ tablespoon Dijon mustard ¼ cup canola oil 1 tablespoon poppy seeds DIRECTIONS Combine all the ingredients in a food processor except for the poppy seeds. Mix in the poppy seeds by hand. Store in a tightly sealed container and keep refrigerated for up to a week.
Sweet Balsamic Dressing	*For six 2-tablespoon servings (per serving: 185 calories; 18 g fat; 0 g of protein; 7 g carbohydrates; 0 g fiber)* 3 tablespoons balsamic vinegar ½ cup olive oil 2 tablespoons honey ½ tablespoon Dijon mustard DIRECTIONS Combine all the ingredients in a food processor. Store in a tightly sealed container and keep refrigerated for several weeks.
Green Secret Sauce	*For eight ¼-cup servings (per serving: 160 calories; 15 g fat; 4 g protein; 4 g carbohydrates; 2 g fiber)* 1 cup tightly packed fresh basil 1 cup tightly packed raw spinach ¼ cup extra-virgin olive oil ¼ cup water ¾ cup raw pine nuts (or raw cashews or raw almonds) ½ tablespoon minced garlic ¼ cup nutritional yeast Heavy pinches of salt and pepper DIRECTIONS Combine all the ingredients in a food processor. Scraping down the processor's sides occasionally, blend until smooth. Store in a tightly sealed container and keep refrigerated for two days.

Salsas and Sauces	Preparation:
Balsamic Reduction	*For two 2-tablespoon servings (per serving: 30 calories; 0 g fat; 0 g protein; 8 g carbohydrates; 0 g fiber)* ½ cup balsamic vinegar DIRECTIONS Pour balsamic vinegar into a small saucepan. Turn the heat to medium high and bring to a boil. Let the balsamic vinegar gently boil for 10 minutes, or until a syrupy liquid forms. Don't overboil or it will become a gel that is impossible to pour.
Carolina BBQ Sauce	*For two ¼-cup servings (per serving: 80 calories; 1 g fat; 1 g protein; 18 g carbohydrates; 1 g fiber)* ¼ cup yellow mustard 1 tablespoon molasses 1 tablespoon honey ½ tablespoon cider vinegar 1 teaspoon chili powder ½ teaspoon cayenne pepper Heavy pinches of dried oregano, salt, and pepper DIRECTIONS Combine all the ingredients in a food processor. Store in a tightly sealed container and keep refrigerated for several weeks.

Lovable Veggies and Side Dishes

Kids are famous for turning up their noses at veggies, but adults scoff at mushy broccoli, too. If you hate vegetables, never fear—you can train your taste buds to actually enjoy healthy fare like carrots, kale, sweet potatoes, collard greens, peas, zucchini, and, yes, even broccoli. Great prepared vegetables are about two things: seasoning and the cooking method. Even the most wonderfully fresh veggie can taste like glue if you overcook and oversalt it. Here are several delicious vegetable and side dishes that will leave you craving more. Yes, really.

Simple Roasted Broccoli

For 2 servings (per serving: 140 calories; 8 g fat; 9 g protein; 16 g carbohydrates; 9 g fiber)

1 head broccoli, rinsed and chopped
1 tablespoon olive or canola oil
¼ tablespoon sea salt
¼ tablespoon pepper

DIRECTIONS

Preheat the oven to 400 degrees.

In a medium bowl, mix the broccoli, oil, salt, and pepper.

Scoop the broccoli evenly onto an oiled cookie sheet and bake for 20 minutes.

Mix It Up: *This simple and versatile recipe also works well with 1-inch pieces of chopped carrots, parsnips, sweet potatoes, Brussels sprouts, and butternut squash.*

Veggie Cheese Bread

For 4 servings (per serving: 135 calories; 5 g fat; 7 g protein; 16 g carbohydrates; 1 g fiber)

4 inches of a whole-grain French bread or other crusty baguette
4 fresh whole basil leaves
½ medium tomato, thickly sliced

½ cup shredded Italian cheese blend (typically a combination of
mozzarella, provolone, Asiago, or other white cheeses)
1 tablespoon minced garlic

DIRECTIONS

Preheat the oven to a low broil.

Slice the baguette into four thin slices.

On each bread slice, layer a basil leaf and one tomato slice. Top with cheese
and a sprinkle of garlic.

Broil for 3–5 minutes, or until the cheese begins to brown.

 ## Caramelized Brussels Sprouts

For 4 servings (per serving: 55 calories; 0.2 g fat; 2 g protein; 13 g carbohydrates;
3 g fiber)

15 Brussels sprouts
2 tablespoons maple syrup
¼ tablespoon sea salt

DIRECTIONS

Preheat the oven to 400 degrees.

Trim the ends off the Brussels sprouts and remove any browning leaves.
Halve any larger sprouts so all are about the same size.

In a small bowl, mix the Brussels sprouts, maple syrup, and sea salt.

Scoop the Brussels sprouts onto an oiled cookie sheet and bake for 20 minutes.

Mix It Up: *Sub in chopped 1-inch pieces of sweet potato and bake for 35 minutes.*

Hummus-Stuffed Mushrooms

For 4 servings (per serving: 60 calories; 3 g fat; 4 g protein; 6 g carbohydrates; 3 g fiber)

12 cremini mushrooms (brown mushrooms with an excellent flavor when roasted) or white mushrooms
½ cup store-bought hummus, any flavor

DIRECTIONS
Preheat the oven to 350 degrees.

Remove the stems from the mushroom caps. Using a wet washcloth, rinse off the caps to remove any dirt.

Spoon a dollop of hummus into each cap, placing the caps hummus-side up on an oiled cookie sheet.

Bake for 25 minutes.

Mix It Up: *Instead of hummus, try stuffing mushroom caps with a drizzle of balsamic vinegar and a large pinch of shredded cheddar cheese. Bake for 25 minutes.*

Simple Steamed Greens

For 2 servings (per serving: 100 calories; 7 g fat; 3 g protein; 7 g carbohydrates; 3 g fiber)

> 1 head kale or collard greens, rinsed and chopped
> ¼ cup water
> 1 tablespoon olive or canola oil
> Salt to taste

DIRECTIONS

Put the greens, water, and oil into a wok.

Cover and turn the heat to medium high.

Steam for 10 minutes, or until the greens have softened.

Pour off any extra liquid and salt to taste.

Better Than Mashed Potatoes

For 4 servings (per serving: 120 calories; 5 g fat; 7 g protein; 14 g carbohydrates; 5 g fiber)

> 1 head cauliflower
> 3 medium parsnips
> ½ cup crumbled goat cheese
> 1 tablespoon fresh parsley, packed
> Salt and pepper to taste

DIRECTIONS

Remove the cauliflower florets from the head.

Peel and chop the parsnips into 1-inch pieces.

In a large saucepan, bring 4 cups of water to a boil. Add the cauliflower and parsnips.

Boil the vegetables until tender but not mushy; approximately 10 minutes. Drain.

In a large bowl, mash together the cauliflower, parsnips, goat cheese, parsley, and salt and pepper. For a creamier texture, use a food processor to combine.

 ## *Collard Greens Coleslaw*

For 4 servings (per serving: 110 calories; 7 g fat; 1 g protein; 12 g carbohydrates; 2 g fiber)

- 1 head collard greens, rinsed well
- ¼ cup red wine vinegar
- 2 tablespoons sugar
- 1 tablespoon Dijon mustard
- 2 tablespoons olive oil
- 1 teaspoon salt
- 2 carrots, peeled and shredded
- ¼ cup shredded red onion

DIRECTIONS

Remove the thick stems from the collard green leaves. Roll the leaves into tight cylinders and slice into thin strips. Roughly chop the strips.

Combine the vinegar, sugar, mustard, oil, and salt in a medium bowl. Stir thoroughly.

Combine the sauce with the collard greens, carrots, and onion. Toss to coat thoroughly.

Chill in the refrigerator for at least an hour, stirring occasionally so the slaw has an even flavor and texture.

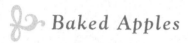 # Baked Apples

For 4 servings (per serving: 110 calories; 3 g fat; 0.2 g protein; 25 g carbohydrates; 3 g fiber)

> 1 tablespoon butter or vegan butter substitute
> 3 apples—2 red (honeycrisp and pink lady are popular) and
>   1 green (Granny Smith is a tart choice)
> 1 tablespoon cinnamon
> 2 tablespoons brown sugar

DIRECTIONS

Preheat the oven to 375 degrees.

Place the butter in the bottom of heavy pie dish and melt it in the oven for a few minutes.

Slice the apples thinly and arrange them in the pie dish. Sprinkle with the cinnamon and brown sugar.

Bake for 45 minutes.

Remove from the oven and let the dish stand for 5 minutes before serving.

Spinach Hummus

For 12 quarter-cup servings (per serving: 115 calories; 4 g fat; 5 g protein;
17 g carbohydrates; 5 g fiber)

2 (15-ounce) cans chickpeas, drained and rinsed
1½ cups packed raw spinach
¼ cup tahini sauce
Juice of one lemon
Two heavy pinches of salt
One heavy pinch of pepper

DIRECTIONS

Combine all ingredients in a food processor and pulse until creamy. This
hummus will keep in the fridge for up to a week.

Holy Deliciousness Bean Dip

For 6 quarter-cup servings (per serving: 125 calories; 6 g fat; 6 g protein;
12 g carbohydrates; 5 g fiber)

1 (15-ounce) can white kidney beans, drained and rinsed
¼ cup goat cheese
1 tablespoon tahini sauce
1 tablespoon fresh rosemary
1 tablespoon olive oil
¼ tablespoon minced garlic
Two heavy pinches of salt
One heavy pinch of pepper

DIRECTIONS

Combine all ingredients in a food processor and pulse until creamy. This dip will keep in the fridge for up to a week.

Smoothies

Depending on the size and ingredients, smoothies are a delicious breakfast, postworkout meal, or simple snack. Smoothies taste best when the fruit is prefrozen, which often eliminates the need to add ice. Buy an extra bunch of ripened organic bananas from the store, peel and slice them, and store in the freezer in a frost-proof plastic bag. You can also buy bags of frozen fruit such as berries and peaches at the grocery store. This is often cheaper than buying fresh fruit and freezing it yourself.

Don't worry if you don't have a fancy blender; it's really more about the order in which you blend the ingredients than the blender itself. Pour in the liquid and yogurt first, and then add the heaviest fruits. Blend for one minute, and then add in the remainder of the ingredients.

Smoothies can also be made ahead of time and stored in airtight containers in the freezer. Let them sit out and thaw for about 30 minutes before drinking. The only disadvantage to making smoothies ahead of time is that the fruit will oxidize and lose some of its nutrients. A light squeeze of fresh lemon juice into your smoothies will help prevent some of the oxidation.

All of the recipes below are for one serving (generally 12 ounces). Additionally, you can add any (or all) of the following mix-ins to each smoothie recipe for an extra nutritional kick:

- **Greens:** Add a handful of raw spinach or kale to a smoothie for an extra dose of vegetables. The greens will turn your smoothie bright green or gray, but I promise—you can't taste it. Try it before you knock it!
- **Omega-3s:** Add a tablespoon of chia seeds or ground flaxseed for a dose of omega-3s.

- **Protein:** To make a smoothie more like a meal and less like a snack, consider adding in two scoops of protein powder. For healthier protein powders, check out pages 135–36.

Berry Smoothie

For 1 serving (per serving: 185 calories; 1 g fat; 10 g protein; 37 g carbohydrates; 5 g fiber)

1 cup milk or milk substitute
½ frozen banana
1 cup frozen mixed berries (you can purchase a package of mixed frozen berries that often include blackberries, blueberries, strawberries, and raspberries)

Nicole's Peanut Butter Shake Smoothie

For 1 serving (per serving: 385 calories; 17 g fat; 25 g protein; 38 g carbohydrates; 3 g fiber)

1 cup milk or milk substitute
3 ounces vanilla yogurt (preferably Greek)
½ banana
2 tablespoons peanut butter
3–5 ice cubes

❧ *Peanut Butter Cup Smoothie*

For 1 serving (per serving: 300 calories; 9 g fat; 21 g protein; 37 g carbohydrates; 3 g fiber)

- 1 cup milk or milk substitute
- 3 ounces vanilla yogurt (preferably Greek)
- ½ frozen banana
- 1 tablespoon peanut butter
- ½ tablespoon cocoa powder

❧ *The Tropics*

For 1 serving (per serving: 290 calories; 16 g fat; 2 g protein; 40 of carbohydrates; 5 g fiber)

- 1 cup light coconut milk
- 1 frozen banana
- ¼ cup packed crushed pineapple

❧ *Peaches and Cream*

For 1 serving (per serving: 260 calories; 0.5 g fat; 17 g protein; 50 g carbohydrates; 3 g fiber)

- 1 cup milk or milk substitute
- 3 ounces vanilla yogurt (preferably Greek)
- ¾ cup frozen peaches
- 1 tablespoon honey or agave nectar
- ½ teaspoon vanilla extract

Angela's Classic Green Smoothie

For 1 serving (per serving: 210 calories; 1 g fat; 12 g protein; 42 g carbohydrates; 4 g fiber)

1 cup milk or milk substitute
2 cups packed raw spinach
1 frozen banana

Creamsicle Smoothie

For 1 serving (per serving: 210 calories; 0.5 g fat; 17 g protein; 35 g carbohydrates; 3 g fiber)

6 ounces vanilla yogurt (preferably Greek)
½ cup orange juice
½ peeled and de-seeded orange
½ teaspoon vanilla extract
3–5 ice cubes

Spicy Chocolate Smoothie

For 1 serving (per serving: 270 calories; 1 g fat; 10 g protein; 60 g carbohydrates; 6 g fiber)

1 cup milk or milk substitute
¼ cup packed dates, pits removed (about 2 large or 4 small dates)
½ cup frozen banana

½ tablespoon cocoa powder
Two heavy pinches of chili powder
Two heavy pinches of ginger

Pumpkin Spice Smoothie

For 1 serving (per serving: 210 calories; 1 g fat; 10 g protein; 42 g carbohydrates;
5 g fiber)

1 cup milk or milk substitute
½ frozen banana
½ cup canned pure pumpkin puree
½ tablespoon maple syrup or agave nectar
½ tablespoon cinnamon
Two heavy pinches of nutmeg

Real-Food Snacks

If you're unprepared, snack time can trip up even the healthiest eater.
When hunger strikes, you *will* tap that vending machine or raid the convenience store for whatever you can find, and it's much more difficult to make
healthy choices when you're already starving.

Here are sixteen healthy snack items to help fuel you in between meals
or after a light workout:

- Two dates slit in half and stuffed with almond butter;
- Celery stuffed with hummus;
- Apple with a slice of cheddar cheese;
- One small handful of nuts;
- Two rice cakes with peanut butter or hummus;

- Greek yogurt and ¾ cup cereal;
- Two cups (measured in the pod) of steamed and lightly salted edamame;
- ½ cup dried apricots;
- Toasted whole wheat pita, cut into triangles and dipped in salsa;
- Glass of orange juice;
- Chopped pear topped with ½ cup cottage cheese;
- Toast with melted cheese;
- Smoothie;
- Whole wheat pretzels dipped in mustard;
- No-Bake Peanut Butter Granola Bar (see recipe below).

Anne's 5-Minute No-Bake Peanut Butter Granola Bars

The following recipe, created by healthy living blogger Anne, yields a dozen healthy, delicious, and affordable bars. Anne has many other healthy, real-food recipes on her site, fANNEtasticFood.com.

For 12 servings (per serving: 190 calories; 7 g fat; 4 g protein; 29 g carbohydrates; 3 g fiber)

DRY (USE SCANT MEASUREMENTS)
1¾ cups oatmeal
1 cup puffed brown rice cereal
¼ cup pumpkin seeds
¼ cup sunflower seeds
¼ cup chia seeds
¼ cup unsweetened coconut
2 tablespoons finely ground flaxseed

WET (USE GENEROUS MEASUREMENTS)
½ cup brown rice syrup
⅓ cup creamy peanut butter
1 teaspoon vanilla extract

DIRECTIONS

Mix all the dry ingredients in a large bowl.

In a microwave-safe medium bowl, blend together the wet ingredients and microwave for 20–30 seconds. (This will make it easier to add the wet ingredients to the dry.)

Pour the wet ingredients into the dry and fold with a spatula until all is well blended.

Pour the mixture evenly into a shallow baking pan and use a spatula to flatten down the mixture. Refrigerate for one hour.

Slice and individually wrap each bar in aluminum foil. Keep in the refrigerator for up to one week.

Part III

EMBRACE STRENGTH

Nine

DEVELOPING AND MAINTAINING AN EXERCISE HABIT

You're too tired. You've never been "sporty." You don't have the time. You have to get to work. You have to go to bed. You have to clean the house. You don't have the energy. You hate the way sweating feels. You can't afford to join a gym.

You just don't feel like it.

Whatever your excuse not to exercise regularly, toss it. Imagine a sheet of paper, with your excuses neatly penned down in a list, and, in your mind's eye, ball up that list and throw it in the trash. Turn to a new, clean sheet of paper. No more excuses this time—let's start again.

You might be a little tired, but you can manage a refreshing walk around the block. You don't have to be naturally athletic to exercise; coming from nothing is *way* more satisfying than being a natural-born speed demon. If you spend even ten minutes a day watching television or surfing the Internet, you also have time to exercise. Energy begets energy; exercise is more effective than drinking coffee. And who said anything about a gym?

Another common story many of us spin about exercise is that it's a chore. You tool around on the stair climber three times a week, but there's no *joy* behind your actions. You have to drag yourself to the weight room or berate yourself into every single run. You think of exercise as one more thing you "must" do. It's not a pleasure; it's an inconvenience on your "to do" list. If you view exercise as a chore, you probably also see it as a form of punishment for "bad" behaviors, like overeating. Exercise may also be a way to smother negative emotions, such as low body confidence or self-esteem. Some people even struggle with *overexercising*, using workouts as a crutch.

Exercise shouldn't ever feel like a chore or a form of punishment. This mind-set sucks all the joy out of exercise. Furthermore, it sets you up to fail and increases the odds that you'll suffer from emotional burnout or a physical injury.

> Don't exercise because you dislike your body. Exercise because you love your body.

Just like we tell ourselves stories about our self-worth ("I'll never be good enough because . . ."), most of us also spin these explanations about why we don't exercise regularly, enjoy exercising, or need to overexercise. The mind is so powerful, and if we tell ourselves these destructive stories for long enough, we start to believe they are infallibly true. If your exercise story is holding you back, physically or emotionally, *you can change your story.* After all, you are the narrator of your own life. If you want a positive, purposeful, and active life, you must begin to think and talk as if you are building a positive, purposeful, and active life.

Small choices add up to amazing results. You can transform your life by waking up each day with the intention to make healthier choices. Perfection is not required. Don't stress out about your goals for next week, next month, or before your big vacation. Focus on today. The only thing you need to do is make a healthy choice *right now.*

Ditch the negative stories you have rolling around in your brain, and focus on creating a new story: "I choose to exercise in a way that inspires me to be healthier, happier, and more confident." Exercise is time to focus on your own physical and emotional needs. It makes you feel and look amazing. It's a break from work, it's fun, it's challenging, it's an excuse to get outside, it motivates you to be healthier in other areas, and it's a way to make new friends. You can learn to embrace exercise, no matter what your current fitness level.

CHOOSING THE HEALTHY OPTION

It really does get easier to make healthy choices over time. Eventually, exercise and healthy cooking will become part of your routine, like brushing your teeth, even if you have to force yourself to do them for the first few months. That's why it's important to focus on small efforts at first. Don't look at it as a complete lifestyle overhaul; being healthy is just a series of choices. Remember, perfection is not the goal. The goal is to make the effort!

Healthy Tipping Point Success Story: Jill, 42, North Carolina

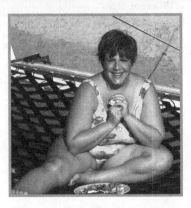 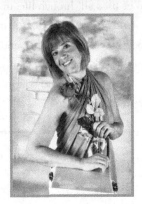

Six years ago, I hit rock bottom. I had a beautiful four-year-old daughter and a loving husband, but I was very depressed. I was on antidepressants, cholesterol medication, and headache medication. I wasted my life away sleeping, eating, crying, and hiding. My depression took so much away from the people I loved the most. I couldn't be a good role model to my daughter or a fun, loving, and spontaneous wife to my husband. I'm not sure what the trigger was for my depression—maybe it was the transition from being a working woman to a full-time mom.

On New Year's Eve, I overheard some friends talking about Weight Watchers, and my friend Jen offered to take me to a meeting and accompany me to the YMCA. I began to take water aerobics classes, but because of my size, I was too embarrassed to do aerobics where I'd need to stand in a studio in front of other people.

I began to make changes bit by bit. First, I just focused on eating my Weight Watcher points, even if I was eating junk. Then, I transitioned to healthier foods. I began to do aerobics, swimming, biking, and running, and I even trained for a sprint triathlon with a group of women from my YMCA. I found it was easy to get stuck in a rut when I exercised alone, but when I did it with friends, I was encouraged to try new things. Eventually, I lost eighty pounds, and my depression lifted.

I have learned that it is okay to be afraid, but I shouldn't be inhibited because of my fears. To be supported and give support is a powerful tool that can be used all through life, in many different areas.

And now I realize that taking care of me is my job, too. My full-time job is being a wife and mother, and that means I have to make myself a priority. I want to take care of my family and be an amazing role model for my daughter. I don't want her to go through the physical or emotional struggles that I went through.

Healthy Tipping Point Exercise FAQs

How Should I Set Fitness Goals?

Expectations are a funny thing. Often, when we decide to change a behavior, we expect to make a 180-degree turn—no matter what negative stories we were just telling ourselves! We expect to be immediately perfect at our new behavior. "I'm going to start exercising," you plot. "I plan to spend an hour in the gym at least five days a week. I will also find time to strength train. Oh, and I will also do yoga before bed three times a week!"

Instead of choosing our goals from the wide spectrum of healthy behaviors between where we are right now and where we want to end up ultimately, we shoot for a total behavior overhaul. Our drastic expectations come from a good place—we're motivated to change and want to tackle our big goals as soon as possible. Unfortunately, this all-or-nothing mentality essentially assures failure.

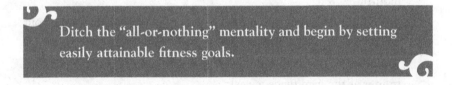

Ditch the "all-or-nothing" mentality and begin by setting easily attainable fitness goals.

In the all-or-nothing world, you're setting yourself up to crash and burn. After all, no one can be perfect, and lifestyle changes are harder to make if you implement many big switches all at once. Small changes, on the other hand, hold firm and build on one another. It's far healthier—and more maintainable—to ditch the all-or-nothing attitude and begin your Healthy Tipping Point journey by setting fitness goals that you can realistically and quickly reach.

MOVE EVERY DAY

Commit to moving your body every day. Don't be intimidated—no one expects (or recommends) that you pound out a hard workout Monday through Sunday. Instead, simply make it your goal to embody one word: *active*. On days that you don't engage in formal exercise, go for a short walk before breakfast, do crunches during commercial breaks, take the stairs instead of the elevator, prepare for bed by doing a few yoga poses, or dance around in your living room while dinner cooks. These little efforts add up and contribute to a more positive attitude about what exercise entails.

Examples of attainable initial fitness goals include:

- Taking a forty-five-minute walk with a neighbor or your dog three times a week.
- Signing up for one new fitness class at the gym every week for a month.
- Stretching every morning with the goal of eventually touching your toes.
- Committing to thirty minutes of strength training with a personal trainer at the gym twice a week.
- Doing a yoga podcast three times a week.
- Training to do fifteen push-ups in a row.

Hopefully, this sample list of initial fitness goals conveys the fact that *something is always better than nothing*. The all-or-nothing mentality is so dangerously toxic. This healthier attitude conveys simple truths: you don't have to be perfect, you can achieve goals, you can integrate new behaviors into your lifestyle, and small efforts really do add up.

You can keep larger, more long-term goals in mind, too—"I want to run a marathon," "I will lose five percent of my body fat," or "I want to make yoga a daily practice." Just don't get so caught up in your long-term goals that you forget to celebrate your short-term achievements, too. The Healthy Tipping Point style of fitness is a lifelong commitment to being active, and everything that happens before and after you reach your long-term goals matters, too.

Remember, your fitness journey is about *health*, not a number on the scale or a race time. If you keep your health in mind, it's easier to make smart decisions about exercise. It's not healthy to skip exercise for weeks on end. It's not healthy to exercise past the point of utter exhaustion. It's not healthy to yo-yo around with your habits, doing nothing and then going full throttle every other month. Healthy exercise is about invigorating your mind and body, reaching your Healthy Ideal, and having fun along the way.

How Much Exercise Is Enough Exercise?

Attainable initial fitness goals are great for boosting confidence and getting into a routine, but what should we be aiming for? How much exercise do you *really* need to be healthy? The answer, according to the Center for Disease Control, depends on how hard you're working.

- 150 minutes a week of moderate-intensity cardiovascular exercise, plus two days of whole-body muscle-strengthening activities;
- 75 minutes a week of high-intensity cardiovascular exercise, plus two days of whole-body muscle-strengthening activities;
- An equivalent combination of moderate- and high-intensity cardiovascular exercise, plus two days of whole-body muscle-strengthening activities. One minute of high-intensity exercise is the same as two minutes of moderate-intensity exercise.[35]

While 150 minutes of exercise might seem like a big chunk of time, you can break it up into manageable little nuggets, like fifteen minutes of brisk walking two times a day, five days a week. Other examples of moderate-intensity exercise include riding a bike, pushing a lawn mower, or doing yoga. Examples of high-intensity exercise include running; swimming; using the elliptical or stair climber at the gym; biking up hills or biking at a rapid pace; or playing sports, like soccer or basketball.

TEN MINUTES OF STRENGTH

Muscle-strengthening activities go beyond lifting weights at the gym; any movement that challenges your muscles through resistance counts. If you don't have access to weights, commit to a ten-minute at-home strength routine two to three times a week. Complete several circuits of push-ups (rest on your knees if you can't do full push-ups yet), sit-ups, planks, squats, and lunges. You can even do your strength routine in front of the TV.

The 150-minute/75-minute recommendation is just the government's minimum for a healthy life. For even greater benefits, engage in close to 300 minutes of moderate-intensity exercise or 150 minutes of high-intensity exercise a week. But you don't want to overdo it, either—there's a point of diminishing returns. More is not always better when it comes to exercise, since putting too much stress on your body can suppress your immune system, cause persistent muscle soreness and body fatigue, delay muscle recovery, overtax your cardiovascular system, trigger amenorrhea (loss of your period), increase your risk of injuries (such as stress fractures or torn tendons), and even impact your mood, causing depression or insomnia.

You cannot—and should not—do it all. When your personal or professional life is stressful, cut back on the intensity and duration of your workouts.

Everyone has a different overdoing-it threshold. One woman may be able to easily pound out 150 minutes of high-intensity training a week. But another woman, who works longer hours or cares for her elderly mother, might feel absolutely knackered after 100 minutes of moderate-intensity exercise and twenty-five minutes of high-intensity exercise a week. You must take into account all the other things going on in your life, too, to find your healthy exercise amount. If you're very busy or stressed, you just might not have the physical energy to expend on lots of high-intensity exercise—as a matter of fact, it might do you more harm than good!

While the attitude of "move your body every day" is a healthy and fun way to get into the exercise habit, rest days from high-intensity exercise are necessary. The importance of these days is often overlooked, seen by some as a useless day away from training, but in reality, they are essential to your training because resting allows your muscles to repair—and grow back stronger. Muscles can take twenty-four to forty-eight hours to fully repair, so you'll want to follow a day of really challenging high-intensity exercise with one day of light stretching. Depending on how your body feels after a day of rest, you may decide to tack on a second day of a short moderate-intensity exercise, like a walk, instead of tackling a hard workout. Exercise should always add to, not subtract from, your energy levels. Other ways to avoid exercise-induced injuries are provided on page 308.

No matter where you're starting or where you want to end up, remember to ease into exercising. Getting into the habit slowly will ensure you stay committed, build your strength and ward off injuries, and prevent mental burnout.

When Should I Exercise?

The best time of day to exercise is . . . whenever you can squeeze it in! There is no ideal time to exercise; working out has a positive impact on your mental and physical health no matter when you do it. That being said, most people have a natural preference for morning or evening workouts.

MORNING VERSUS EVENING WORKOUTS

Morning Workout Advantages	Evening Workout Advantages
You won't blow off your workout if the day gets too busy. Working out in the morning starts the day off with a healthy habit.	You get to sleep in longer.
Working out in the morning helps some people wake up.	Some find they naturally have more energy at night.
In the warmer months, outdoor exercise is more comfortable in the early morning.	Many people find it easier to eat proper portions throughout the day if they exercise at night.
Some people find evening exercise makes it harder to fall asleep.	Other people find evening exercise is a relaxing way to wind down.

Your body and your schedule are unlike anyone else's. It's really a matter of figuring out what works best for *you*. If you do choose to work out in the morning, you'll want to time your breakfast carefully to ensure you have the fuel you need to power through your workout—but don't hurl it back up all over your sneakers. Check out page 254 for information on fueling your workouts.

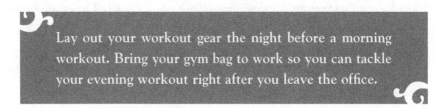

Lay out your workout gear the night before a morning workout. Bring your gym bag to work so you can tackle your evening workout right after you leave the office.

How Can I Stay Motivated?

The hardest part of integrating exercise into your daily life isn't getting started—it's keeping the habit going! Staying motivated can be a challenge, and it's helpful to remember that everyone's motivation levels naturally ebb and flow. One week, you'll kick butt at your workouts. The next, you might have to drag yourself out of bed. This is completely normal. The trouble, of course, occurs when you experience an ebb and don't ever get back into the flow.

To stay motivated over the long haul, try these simple tricks:

- **Plan Your Workouts in Advance:** At the beginning of each week, pencil (or type) your workouts into your calendar. Stop thinking of exercise as "optional" and consider it "me time" that you cannot miss. This technique ensures you'll find the time to fit in your 75 or 150 minutes of high- or moderate-intensity exercise a week. For example, if you plan in advance, you'll realize that you *have* to exercise in the morning on Tuesday because you have a late meeting that night.

  Alternatively, you can plan out a week's worth of workouts but not tie them to a specific day. This technique is helpful if you have a flexible schedule or prefer not to be so rigid in your healthy habits.

- **Keep Track of Your Completed Workouts:** Remember when you were in kindergarten and you got a gold star every time you completed a task? Apply the same small-rewards mentality to your daily workouts. Keep track of what you did, even if it's something small; looking back over several weeks of effort will boost your confidence and help keep you on track. You can write your workouts on a calendar on the fridge, create a spreadsheet on your computer, tick off the workouts in your planner, keep track on your smartphone, or even actually give yourself little gold star stickers for every active day. When you reach a certain milestone, give yourself a reinforcing reward, as discussed on pages 37–38 of the "Get Real" section.

> Exercise should add to, not detract from, your overall energy levels.

- **Give It Ten:** You can do anything for ten minutes. If you're feeling lazy and would rather flop down on the couch than sweat, commit to exercising for just ten minutes. After ten minutes, you can happily reacquaint yourself with the couch. Odds are, however, that you'll stick with your workout until the end.

- **Better Together:** Enlist your partner, a friend, or a coworker as your exercise pal. Studies show that workout buddies hold each other accountable; even virtual workout buddies—through e-mails, blogs, or even video games—can increase motivation.[36] If you agree to meet your pal at 7 a.m. for a run, you won't keep hitting that snooze button—someone else is waiting for you! Buddies can also help you get over workout embarrassment and encourage you to try new activities, since you'll have someone to talk to and learn from.

It's important to pick the *right* kind of buddy. You want an exercise pal who will motivate and inspire you, not hold you back. That doesn't mean they have to be at the exact same fitness level as you. If you're helping someone else get started, you can use your joint workouts as easy days and go harder when working out alone. But, steer clear of workout buddies who are emotionally toxic or flake out on you too often.

A great place to find new exercise buddies is at the gym. It's normal to feel awkward when you first start taking exercise classes, like Zumba or yoga, because it can feel like everyone else knows one another already. The majority of exercise classes are very welcoming, friendly, and not judgmental (if yours seems too cliquey, try another studio!). Introduce yourself to the instructor on the first day and explain you're a newbie. If you continue to come back, people will begin to recognize your smiling face and see you as a regular, too.

If you can't find any real-life buddies, find some online—there are literally millions of potential buddies out there. Check out a healthy online community like SparkPeople.com, Livestrong.com, or DailyMile.com.

"I'M EMBARRASSED!"

Many people are embarrassed to exercise in front of others because they're "too big," "too old," "too clumsy," "too stupid," or just "too nervous." In fact, in one nationwide study, one-third of all respondents said they were too intimidated to exercise at the gym.[37] Letting fear control you is no way to reach your Healthy Tipping Point! Whenever you are nervous, repeat this mantra: "Everyone is a beginner at some point, and it is okay not to be perfect. My workouts are for me."

Yes, people might watch you during an exercise class, at the gym, or as you jog down the road, but odds are high that they're admiring your tenacity, wondering where you got your shirt, or simply staring into space—not mentally tearing you up. Most people are so wrapped up in their own workout that they're not wasting time criticizing others. And if they *are* judging you . . . well, they're negative, no-good energy vampires. Why let people like that impact your happiness?

Workout buddies are one effective way to get over exercise embarrassment. Smaller, local gyms can be less intimidating than larger, "cooler" gyms (and they're also usually cheaper!). If you're confounded by workout equipment, ask a trainer at the gym to show you how to use it; there is no shame in asking! No one knows what to do the first time they step on a treadmill. If you're nervous about taking an exercise class, simply pop your head in and check out the class before you attend. Certain classes, like introductory yoga and Zumba, are notoriously welcoming. Buying properly fitting workout clothes, including a supportive sports bra and compression capris, will also help you feel more comfortable. And last, remember this: you're awesome and inspiring for tackling your fears. If you can do this, you can do anything.

If you want to change your life, you must let go of fear. Failure is never trying.

- **Bust Through Plateaus:** A plateau is simply a euphemism for a rut. If you do the same exercise over and over again, your body becomes highly proficient at the movements and, thus, doesn't have to work as hard. If you're steadily losing weight for weeks on end, and then the scale doesn't budge for a month, you're likely plateauing. Plateaus also impact your cardiovascular and muscular fitness. If you run the same pace every time, you'll never get faster. And sometimes, a plateau is all in your head—you're bored with the same old workouts.

  To bust through physical and mental plateaus, do something new. Challenge your body with an interval workout (check out page 291 for examples), lift heavier weights, or try an entirely new activity. If you're struggling with a weight-loss plateau, your diet may be to blame; go back to the basics—clean eating, portion control, and listening to hunger cues—for several weeks to see if there's an improvement.

- **Race!:** If you're struggling to stay motivated, sign up for a race. Yes—a *real* race. You can train for a 5K (3.1 miles) in eight weeks using a walk/run method (see the Start-from-Scratch Walk/Run Training Plan on page 317) or you can aim higher and do a 10K, half-marathon, or even a full marathon. America's passion for racing continues to grow—in 1976, 25,000 Americans did a marathon; the number exploded to 507,000 by 2010[38]—and people of all ages and fitness levels are getting involved. Racing isn't just for high school kids at track meets; most racers are in their late thirties and early forties. Racing is tremendously fun, and if you look at the event as a celebration of training, signing up (and paying that race entry fee) can help keep you motivated and focused.

How Should I Fuel My Workouts?

Food is fuel for your body, and when your machine is working extra hard—such as during exercise—it's paramount that you not only get *the right amount and type* of fuel but that you also fuel at *the right time*. "How should

I fuel my workouts?" is a simple question with a very complex answer. What you should eat, how much you should eat, and when you should eat varies greatly according to your workout, your fitness or weight-loss goals, your age, and your body type.

> Commit to taking a fifteen-minute walk at the same time of day, every day. This healthy habit adds up to 105 minutes of exercise each week!

Splitting Meals

Your body uses energy from the food you've recently consumed, as well as stored carbohydrates (known as glycogen, which is stored in your liver, fat cells, and muscles) to power through activity. When engaging in light exercise (both in duration and intensity), you probably do not need to eat *specifically* for the workout. You're only burning a (relatively) small amount of calories, which your body has easy access to, assuming that your overall calorie intake is nutritious and adequate.

That being said, many people find that exercising on an empty stomach is miserable. Some may experience blood sugar drops if energy from food isn't readily available. Others may feel weak and easily fatigued without something in their stomach. But stuffing yourself with a big meal right before you hit the gym isn't ideal, either. If your stomach is still digesting food, you'll experience cramping and nausea during the workout.

By splitting meals into pre- and postworkout minimeals, you can avoid the unpleasant side effects associated with eating too much, too little, too late, or too soon during light exercise.

For example, let's say you prefer to exercise in the morning. When you wake up, you're already a little hungry (after all, you haven't eaten for eight to ten hours!), but if you eat your entire breakfast right away, you have to wait an hour before exercising or you get cramps. On the other hand, if you held off on breakfast and went straight to your workout, by the time your one-hour yoga class was over, you'd be gnawing the edge of your mat. The solution is to split breakfast into breakfast number one and breakfast number two, each a minimeal that provides your body with the specific pre- and postworkout nutrients it needs to perform and recover. The same theory can be applied to midday workouts. If you like to exercise during your lunch break but are already hungry by the time you make it to the gym, have a small snack—lunch number one—before exercising and follow up with lunch number two, which would be more filling.

Alternatively, you can time your snacks around your workout. If it's most convenient to exercise right after work, eat a small snack around four or five o'clock.

For moderate to strenuous exercise (both in duration and intensity), simply splitting meals will not be enough. You'll need extra fuel—calories—for your workouts. You can get these calories by eating during exercise, eating larger meals, or eating more snacks. More information about fueling for endurance exercise is provided below.

THE BEST PRE- AND POSTWORKOUT FUEL

The best preworkout fuel is high in carbohydrates but relatively low in protein and fat, which digest more slowly than carbohydrates and can upset the stomach during exercise. Examples include a slice of toast with a smear of peanut butter, fruit juice, whole-grain cereal with skim milk or milk substitute, or cooked oatmeal with a banana. The size of your preworkout fuel will vary depending on what else you've eaten that day, your size, and the intensity and duration or your workout. If you experience symptoms of hunger during your workout, you may need to eat more beforehand or supplement with midworkout fuel (see "A Note About Moderate to Intense Exercise" on the facing page).

The best postworkout fuel contains carbohydrates, protein, and fat. Protein is especially important for muscle recovery. Examples include rice, beans, and vegetables; a smoothie made with nut butter; or an egg and cheese sandwich on whole wheat bread. Again, the size of your postworkout fuel will vary. It's important to eat as soon as possible—aim for within a half hour—following a hard workout. Otherwise, your body will feast on itself, breaking down muscle tissue to replenish energy.

A Note About Moderate to Intense Exercise

If you're engaging in moderate to intense exercise—working out four to six days a week—you'll need to pay special attention to your diet to ensure you do not under- or overeat. If you undereat, you're putting yourself at risk for mental and physical burnout. Chronically underfueling can trigger acute injuries, such as stress fractures; cause long-term damage to your body; and hamper performance. On the other hand, if you overeat, your body will store the extra fuel as body fat. It is surprisingly easy to overeat—even when training for an event like a marathon—because we tend to overestimate how hard we're working.

Striking the right balance between a healthy diet and an active lifestyle can be challenging. To hit that sweet spot of ideal fueling, follow these tips.

- **Eat More:** On days you exercise more than usual, you should also eat more food. You'll want to eat back any *extra* calories you burned if you want to maintain your weight. For example, let's say you normally run three miles three times a week but work up to five miles three times a week. If you burn an extra 150–200 calories (depending on your size) by adding two miles to your workout regimen, you'll need to eat an *additional* 150–200 calories on the days you run to maintain your starting weight. While two more miles feels like a lot of extra work, 150–200 calories is only equal to two slices of dry toast.

  It can be difficult to eat back your exercise calories in one day, especially if you begin to compete in endurance events, like long-distance running, and are committed to eating real, plant-based foods.

It's not necessary to stuff yourself—your refueling can continue the next day with a slightly larger breakfast or an extra snack.

- **Do a Count Check-In:** Consider occasional count check-ins to assess your eating habits and ensure you're eating the correct amount of food. Whether you calorie count on your longest workout day, once a week, or once a month, such check-ins can really help you stay on track with balanced eating habits. The Harris Benedict equation on page 125 will give you a rough idea of how much you should be eating to maintain your weight and health while participating in moderate to intense exercise. Additionally, below is a list of estimated calorie burns for thirty minutes of different types of exercise, for a 150-pound person.

Remember that a lot of calorie counting is really just fuzzy math. No machine or chart knows for sure how much you burned, and it's impossible to know exactly how much you're eating. The purpose of count check-ins isn't to make you feel restricted, guilty, or obsessive; the check-ins will just give you a very rough idea of whether you're refueling properly.

CALORIES BURNED DURING THIRTY MINUTES OF EXERCISE

Activity	Calories Burned	Activity	Calories Burned
Aerobics, low impact	200	Rowing, moderate effort	240
Bicycling, casual pace	135	Running, six miles per hour	340
Bicycling, moderate pace	270	Stair climber, moderate effort	300
Dancing, moderate effort	200	Swimming, light effort	215
Elliptical trainer, hard effort	390	Walking, casual pace	110
Jogging, moderate pace	240	Weight lifting, light effort	100
Pilates, moderate effort	175	Yoga, high effort (hot yoga)	240
Racquetball	240	Yoga, light effort	100

Note: All calories estimates assume a 150-pound person.

- **Follow Hunger Cues:** It's especially important to listen to your hunger cues, since signs of weakness or fatigue after training can indicate that you're underfueling. Golden rule? If you're hungry in between meals, eat! Have a healthy snack that includes complex carbohydrates, protein, and fat (check out pages 236–38 for examples) and drink a large glass of water.
- **Fuel During Training:** If you find that you are especially hungry following moderate to intense exercise, you may need to eat *during* training. Midexercise snacks are ideal—and often necessary—for people exercising at a high level for more than an hour. Providing your body with a constant source of carbohydrates will keep your energy up. Take in thirty to sixty grams of easily digestible carbohydrates (120–240 calories) every hour. If you're planning to exercise for an extended period of time—say, you're doing a long bike ride—don't wait until two hours into the ride to start fueling! The calories you consume during exercise should, of course, be factored into your overall caloric intake for the day.

  Sports gels, such as Clif Shots or Hammer Gel, are popular fueling options for runners and cyclists. These 80–100-calorie packets contain simple carbohydrates (sugars) that athletes can simply squirt into their mouths. Sport gels are also sold in solid form, as jelly beans or fruit chews. Sport gels, while convenient to carry and eat, are expensive and usually contain fake-food products. Natural alternatives to gels include dates, packets of honey, raisins, and pieces of whole fruit. Stick 'em in a plastic bag and safety pin the bag to the inside of your shorts if you don't have a pocket.

  It's important to drink water during all durations and intensities of exercise, but it's equally imperative that you drink water when fueling. Water will help your body digest the food and convert it into energy. If you're exercising in the heat or sweating excessively, you should also drink an electrolyte-replacement beverage, such as Gatorade or coconut water. Seek out the regular, full-calorie Gatorade; the low-calorie version is made with artificial sweeteners and doesn't offer a significant source of carbohydrates. If you opt for coconut water, an all-natural alternative to Gatorade, remember that it is relatively low in calories, and you'll need to supplement with additional fuel.

If you're exercising for less than an hour and are not sweating excessively, you probably do not need to consume calories or drink anything besides water during exercise.

• **Don't Fill Up on Empty Calories:** While a healthy diet certainly has room for treats—whether you're exercising or not—it's unwise to refuel entirely with empty calories for several reasons. It is *extremely* easy to go overboard on empty calories following hard exercise. Very often, people view exercise as a free pass to eat whatever they want. It's all too easy to overestimate how much we burned off and underestimate the size of treats. Many marathon runners, for example, actually gain weight during training simply because they overeat in response to their rigorous training.

Furthermore, if your body is working hard, it needs more *nutrients*—not just more calories! Your body is craving the inflammation-fighting, tissue-repairing nutrients found in healthy foods, including whole grains, healthy fats, fruits and vegetables, plant-based proteins, dairy, nuts and seeds, and other lean proteins. Filling up on wholesome, plant-based foods will ensure a faster recovery, ward off injuries, and keep your energy levels sky-high. Balance the occasional scoop of ice cream with a serving of veggies, and you'll be just fine.

A Note About Weight Loss

In the "But What About Calories?" discussion on page 122, we addressed how exercise increases your caloric needs. This topic is worth revisiting here. The more often and harder you exercise, the more fuel you need to power through and recover after workouts. When you burn more calories than you take in through food, your body utilizes its most readily available energy stores—body fat or, secondarily, muscle—for fuel. Therefore, if you want to increase your exercise but maintain your body weight, you need to replace the calories you burn through extra fuel. If you want to lose weight, you must create a *small* calorie deficit each day from exercise and/or diet. But you *never* want to create a severe calorie deficit, since eating too little and exercising too hard is extremely dangerous and can trigger a host of physical and emotional problems.

Slow and steady always wins the race when it comes to weight loss—crash dieting, underfueling, and excessive exercise is the exact opposite of a Healthy Tipping Point. This behavior is not maintainable, healthy, or safe.

HUNGRY OR THIRSTY?

People often mistake thirst for hunger. Aim to drink half of your weight in pounds in ounces of water each day. If you eat many plants, which naturally contain water, you may need to drink less water. If you exercise, you will likely need to drink more.

When you're losing weight through diet and exercise, it can be difficult to tell the difference between "good" hunger and "bad" hunger. If you create a deficit of 250 calories a day (a safe and maintainable amount for weight loss) through diet and exercise, you will naturally feel a little hungrier than you did before. After all, your belly—although it's filled with *enough* high-quality food, especially if you focus on eating nutrient-dense plant foods—is filled with *less* food. Signs of bad hunger include dizziness, nausea, irritability, sleepiness, growling stomach, sudden weight loss, headaches, and irregular bowel movements/constipation. If you experience any of these symptoms in between meals, eat a snack immediately. Ignoring bad hunger signs will only cause health problems down the road.

Healthy Tipping Point Success Story: Simon, 29, United Kingdom

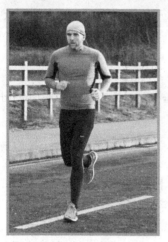

I've been blind since I was eighteen. I have retinitis pigmentosa, a degenerative eye disease that attacks the retina and destroys its ability to process images before sending information to the brain. Being blind introduces a number of challenges in my daily life; certain tasks can be completed only with support or guidance. I won't bore you with the psychological effects and the stressors involved. I will just say it's stressful.

My level of fitness has generally been dictated by the assistance that I can receive. I could only run as fast as my guide runners could run or push as hard as my friends at the gym could go. I never felt having a guide held me back in any way, but it did create a link between our fitness levels.

In the middle of 2010, I lost all of my guide runners and workout buddies. I sat in my living room, pondering how I could return to some kind of activity. Of all the sports, running seemed like the best bet. But I couldn't afford a treadmill or gym membership, so running on my own was my only option.

I persuaded my wife to take me to a closed road near to our house. With no pedestrians and cars, it was the perfect training ground for me. I ran on the closed road for a number of weeks until I became bored. Running for long distances on a .15-mile closed road is mind-numbingly boring. I felt I had come this far, so why not just venture out onto the road? I decided to just go for it, stepped out onto the road, and just ran. Over the coming months, I spent my time memorizing the road surfaces, learning the camber of the path, and pairing the information with audio-based GPS markers. Using this technique, I memorized a three-mile route and ran it regularly.

With my fitness level back up to where it was before my break, I needed another challenge to conquer.

For my first-ever race, I chose to run the Cotswold 100 Ultra—a hundred-mile race. I felt this would push me both mentally and physically, which was my main focus. I ended up pushing myself eighty-three miles, and then I had to pull out. The race was amazing but grueling, and after eighty-three miles, I literally could no longer support my own body weight—my legs, but not my spirit, gave out on me. The Cotswold 100 was just the beginning of my ultramarathon career; I can't wait to tackle and complete other races.

Self-belief is the driving force of what I do. In all of us, there is the possibility of change. We can all achieve great fitness goals if we simply believe in ourselves. There will always be setbacks—some small, like a missed turn during a race, and some large, like my blindness—but these setbacks simply lay a foundation for future success. Life is about picking yourself back up, believing, and moving forward.

Ready, Set, Gear Up!

Remember how it felt to organize your new notebooks and markers on the first day of school? Just for a brief (very brief) moment, you were actually psyched that summer was over and classes were beginning—heck, you had a shiny pencil case to play with!

Exercise gear is the adult version of a pencil case. There's something exciting—and tremendously motivating—about a new workout top, perfect sneakers, or a pass to a different exercise class. Well-fitting gear also makes exercise more comfortable, enjoyable, and safe.

Does this mean you need to spend hundreds of dollars on designer yoga pants? Absolutely not. The key to quality gear is finding clothing and equipment that works for *your body shape*, which does not necessarily mean the most expensive type.

GET THRIFTY

Discount department stores and big-box retailers offer high-quality workout gear and shoes at rock-bottom prices. You might have to scour the racks, but you can walk away with great deals, like sweat-wicking tops for ten dollars or less! Additionally, save extra dough by shopping for out-of-season gear. You'll save money by stocking up on long-sleeve shirts in the summer and shorts in the winter.

Workout Clothing

Ditch the cotton clothes and invest in some sweat-wicking tops, bottoms, and sport bras. This fabric helps keep you dry and cool by transferring sweat away from your body and toward the outside of the fabric. It is also more breathable than cotton or other synthetic fabrics, so you sweat less to begin with.

There are many options when it comes to workout tops: sleeveless, sleeved, short, long, baggy, tight, with a bra shelf or without. The best type of top is whatever you feel more comfortable and confident in. Similarly, there's a variety of workout bottoms—shorts, shorts with underwear built in, capris, flared pants, tight pants, skin-tight shorts—and you should purchase whatever works for you. If you experience chafing (which is when your skin rubs against another body part or clothing and burns) between your legs, purchase a pair of skintight spandex shorts. You can wear the shorts under baggy shorts if you wish, but the tight spandex will prevent thigh burn.

When exercising outdoors, dress as if it is twenty degrees warmer.

If you're exercising outside, you'll also need to consider gear for the heat and the cold. Dress as if it's twenty degrees warmer. If the thermometer says it's sixty degrees, it's going to feel like eighty once you start sweating. If it's thirty, you won't be chilly for long! For warm weather, a sweat-wicking hat will help shade your face while allowing your head to breathe. Dressing for cold weather is a bit more complicated. It's just as important to wear sweat-wicking clothing in cold weather; the fabric will keep your skin dry, thereby helping to maintain body temperature. You'll want to dress in layers so you can take off clothing as you warm up. For a chilly run, you'll probably need winter running tights, a sweat-wicking undershirt, a sweat-wicking pullover or long-sleeve shirt, gloves, and earmuffs or a hat.

For the majority of women, the most important piece of exercise gear is undoubtedly the sports bra. After all, the breasts have little natural support—only skin and thin ligaments—and the movement created by exercise can be incredibly painful. In fact, research suggests that breasts move an average of ten centimeters—almost four inches—during vigorous exercise. Women with larger breasts experience even more movement. And breasts don't just move up and down; they also swing side to side, creating a very uncomfortable figure-eight pattern.[39]

The first sports bra was two jockstraps sewn together. Thankfully, sports-bra design has progressed by leaps and bounces since the late 1970s. A high-quality sports bra restricts breast movement in all directions, preventing breast pain, back pain, and chafing. In addition to physical comfort, a well-fitted sports bra also provides a sense of modesty, which can reduce feelings of exercise embarrassment and allow you to more fully focus on your workout.

Here are a few tips for finding the perfect sports bra to house your puppies:

- Skip the online stores and try on bras for the best fit. Shop in specialty athletic stores, since they'll offer a wider variety of high-quality bras designed especially for high-impact exercise.

- Sports bras come in two general designs: compression and encapsulation. Compression bras, which literally compress your breasts against your chest, are thought to be more effective for smaller cup sizes (A and B). Encapsulation bras surround and support each breast separately and are more effective for larger cup sizes (C and higher). Encapsulation bras may also come with underwire for added support. If you have larger breasts, seek out sport bras that are sized by cup sizes; you'll get a better all-around fit with these than with bras sized small, medium, or large.
- Select sports bras made with sweat-wicking material, because cotton bras will get wet and stretch as you exercise.
- If you have a larger chest, select sport bras with wide shoulder straps that crisscross in the back (racerback); this design will take pressure off your shoulders.
- The best sports bra is not necessarily the tightest. A sports bra shouldn't restrict your breathing or cut into your skin.
- Jog in place in the dressing room to test out the bounce control. If the elastic band of the bra moves up when you lift your arms above your head, it's too loose around your rib cage. Last, double-check the seams and closures of the bra for rough edges that would trigger chafing.

SWEATY STENCH, GO AWAY!

To get that sweaty stench out of your workout clothes, add a quarter-cup baking soda to your regular detergent. Washing workout clothes separately and in small loads will also help remove the odor of all your hard work. To ensure your workout clothing lasts as long as possible, wash on the coldest setting for delicate fabrics and never, ever put your gear in the dryer. Skip the fabric softener or dryer sheet, since the chemicals in softeners actually interfere with the sweat-wicking properties of your gear. Air-drying your gear helps it last longer.

Athletic Shoes

Interesting (and slightly scary) fact: when you're running and your foot strikes the ground, the impact force inflicted on your body is two to three times your body weight.[40] Over the course of a mile, you'll strike the ground around 1,000 times! This high-impact force can wreak havoc on your joints, bones, and muscles, so it is absolutely imperative that you invest in a pair of well-fitted athletic shoes if you plan to do any type of walking, running, aerobics, or other impact-based exercise.

There are many "rules" about sneaker replacement. Some runners swear that shoes must be replaced every 300 miles. Others believe in tossing out the kicks after 500 miles. And some wait until the shoes literally begin to fall apart. But the best guideline is to go by how your legs feel—if your muscles, shins, or knee joints begin to feel unusually achy after exercise, it's a sure sign that the cushioning has worn out, and the sneakers need to be replaced.

When it comes to selecting a running shoe, it's not enough to ask your active friends, "What type of shoe do you wear?" Your feet and gait are unique, and different shoes work for different people. Head over to a specialty running store or athletic store and speak to an educated salesperson about your goals and activity level. Also, ask about the return policy; many specialty stores will let you return shoes—even if you've worn them—if they don't work out.

There are several issues to consider when seeking a sneaker:

- **Your Sport:** Different activities require different shoes. If you plan to walk, you'll want to shop for a special walking shoe. If you plan to run, you'll need a running shoe. And if you plan to do aerobics or dance—well, there's a shoe for that, too! Each type of shoe is designed especially to protect your feet from the exact movements of the sport. If you're just looking for a shoe for general gym work, try a running shoe.
- **Your Arch:** Do you have a high arch, a normal arch, or flat feet? Take the wet test; you'll need a shallow pan of water and two pieces of paper. Step in the water in your bare feet, and then step on and off

the paper. Your footprint shape will reveal your arch type. If you can see your entire footprint, you have flat feet or a low arch. If you can only see the ball of your foot, your heel, and a thin streak connecting the two, you have a high arch. If your footprint shows half your arch, you have a normal arch.

> Shop for athletic shoes late in the day—when your feet are naturally swollen—and buy half a size to a size larger than your dress shoe size.

- **Your Foot Stability:** If you have a low arch, you most likely pronate: during a foot strike, your arch collapses and your ankle rolls in. If you have a high arch, you may supinate: your ankle rolls out during a foot strike. You may also have a normal arch and experience pronation or supination, but it's more likely that you run with a neutral form. Your foot may roll in slightly, but the rest of your leg—particularly your knee joint—stays in position. Sneakers come with varying degrees of motion control and cushioning to minimize the negative impact of pronation and supination.
- **Your Size:** Don't base your athletic shoe size on your dress-shoe size—you'll need at least half a size to a size larger because your feet will swell during activity.

BAREFOOT IS BEST?

Barefoot running is incredibly cool—but is it safe? The minimalist movement, popularized by Christopher McDougall's book *Born to Run* and the Vibram FiveFingers minimalist shoe, contends that humans were designed to run and regular sneakers interfere with proper biomechanics. However, the research on minimalist running is inconclusive; some reports say barefoot running reduces injuries, and others argue that the practice exacerbates bad form.

If you do decide to try minimalist shoes, it's extremely important that you break them in over several months—start off with five minutes a day, three times a week and *very* gradually increase your distance.

All runners can take one lesson away from the minimalist movement: land softly and avoid heel striking, which is when you land on your heel. Paying attention to your gait will reduce impact and ward off injuries.

Other Workout Investments

You've got clothes on your back and sneakers on your feet—so what else do you need to exercise? Truthfully, not much. You can become healthier by walking, jogging, or running around your neighborhood for free. Everything else—the special water bottles, the iPod, the no-slip headbands—are just extras. Just like any hobby, when it comes to exercise gear, there's always *something* else you could buy.

Here are just a few of the extras.

- **Gym Membership:** Choose a gym that's close to your home or work and is open well past the hours you plan to attend—or you'll never make it. Ask for a free weeklong pass to the gym so you can ensure it's your scene and you feel comfortable. Remember that employees have a membership sales quota to reach every week or month; gym prices are always negotiable! A long-term contract might help you feel more committed, but it can also be tremendously inconvenient—your life might change, and you may end up working or living far from the gym. Don't get locked into a long-term contract if you can help it.
- **Exercise Classes:** You can find exercise classes at the gym or in specialty studios. Most studios offer a free class to new students. Ask the

front-desk attendant which class is best for beginners and who are the most popular instructors. At the beginning of the class, go ahead and introduce yourself as a new student to the instructor. A great instructor will assist and encourage you without embarrassing you in front of the group. If you're not feeling a particular class is a match, don't assume that you just don't like yoga or Zumba—it might be the studio or instructor, not the activity. Give it a few more tries or try a different class before giving up.

> If you frequently travel for work, pack a workout DVD and exercise in your hotel room.

- **Workout DVDs:** Workout DVDs are a convenient, cheap alternative to joining a gym or studio. DVDs also allow you to exercise right in your living room, so they're a great option during the winter or for people with small children. There are so many inspiring DVDs, and new ones come out all the time, but a few great options include *30 Day Shred* by Jillian Michaels and *Bob Harper: Yoga for the Warrior* by Bob Harper.
- **Hydration Belts/Backpacks:** Hydration belts and backpacks keep you hydrated—and your hands free. Hydration belts clip around the waist and include four or six small water bottles. Hydration backpacks—such as the popular CamelBak—hold a water bladder with a long, flexible straw. Many backpacks hold at least one and a half quarts of water.
- **Safety Gear:** When it comes to outdoor exercise, the most effective piece of safety gear is . . . common sense. Stay alert, carry a cell phone, tell other people where you'll be going and when you should be back, avoid dark alleys and deserted parking lots, and carry identification and emergency contact information. You can even get engraved

bracelets or dog tags so you don't have to worry about carrying a license—Road ID is one popular brand (roadid.com). If you like to listen to music, turn the volume down or wear one ear bud. Wear a reflective vest or a blinking light if you exercise at dawn or dusk. Most important, vary your exercise routes—it's tempting to walk or run the same path over and over again, but it establishes a pattern that criminals can take advantage of.

There are also a variety of protection devices, such as pepper spray or whistles, for sale at specialty running stores or online.

STOP THAT DOG

If you exercise in rural areas, odds are high that you'll eventually encounter a territorial, unchained dog. When a dog running loose approaches you, assume a nonthreatening stance—look down, don't show your teeth, turn your body to the side, and tuck your hands in your armpits or clench your fists to protect your fingers. In a deep, confident voice, tell the dog to go home.

If the dog continues to advance, begin to slowly back away, scanning the ground for large rocks or sticks that can be used as a weapon in case the dog attacks. Alternatively, you can use your leg to block an approach. If the dog attacks and you cannot get away, protect your face and try to use your body weight to pin the dog to the ground. Always report aggressive dogs on the loose to animal control; you're doing other runners and neighborhood children a favor!

- **Music:** Studies show that listening to music while exercising can reduce your perception of how difficult the workout feels by as much as 10 percent.[41] So rock it out! There are armband and waist-clip attachments for iPods and other music devices. Make sure you're safe with your music—never turn it up so high that you can't hear the outside world. Again, if you're exercising outside, turn down the music or use only one ear bud. Never listen to music while riding a bicycle since you are sharing the road or path with other traffic, including runners and cars. Last, remember not to push yourself too hard; sometimes, we get caught up in the beat and forget to listen to our body.

> Swap motivating playlists with your workout buddy so you always have new, energizing tunes.

- **Bicycle and Indoor Trainer:** There are three general types of bicycles: mountain bikes (heavy, sturdy frames and very thick tires); road bikes (light frames and very skinny tires); and hybrid bikes (medium frames and medium tires). Mountain bikes are, of course, suited for mountain biking; they are built to go over rocks and sticks. Hybrid bikes are a good choice for casual riding around the city. And road bikes are designed for long distances or race situations, like triathlons. Generally speaking, mountain bikes are cheaper than road bikes. You can buy a new bike—at a local bike shop—or seek out a used bike online. If you're buying used, it's still a good idea to head to the bike shop first to determine what size bike you'll need (don't feel bad about just browsing—you'll be back with your used bike for a tune-up!). Always visibly inspect a used bike before purchasing it; check for cracks in the frame, since this is a very expensive problem to fix. Rusty chains or old tires are relatively cheap to replace. If the seller is shipping your used bike to you from far away, ask for close-up photographs of the entire frame.

  Once you've got your bike, consider buying an indoor trainer. This device allows you to turn your bike into a stationary bike so you can ride year-round, no matter what the weather!

Healthy Tipping Point Success Story: Linda, 51, Maryland

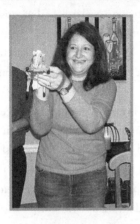 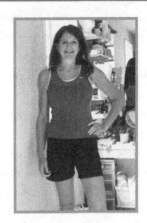

A little more than ten years ago, I went on a medication that caused me to gain thirty-five pounds. A few years later, I developed high blood pressure and high cholesterol from the extra weight, poor eating habits, and lack of exercise. My cardiologist laid it all out on the line for me: I either had to lose weight or go on medication for my blood pressure and cholesterol. I decided not to take the "easy" route with medication.

Instead of crash dieting, I decided to truly get *healthier*—I started walking, taking long, fast walks through my neighborhood. It was kind of enjoyable! I was starting to eat a larger variety of foods and watching my portion sizes. I was still eating processed and pre-prepared foods, but the weight was coming off—slowly but surely.

Then, I signed up for the Montgomery County Road Runners Club's Beginning Women's Running program. Runners are the most welcoming people in the world. They don't care if you are fast or slow or can't even run a mile; they just want to support each other. The group taught me a lot about running—how to train, what to wear, and what to do about injuries. Running motivated me to focus on better nutrition and eating habits. I stopped eating processed foods, bought organic fruits and vegetables, and started keeping track of my diet and exercise habits so I would have a clearer idea of what I was doing right and what areas I needed to work on.

That summer, I showed up at the cardiologist's office at my goal weight. He was shocked. I imagine he gives everyone a goal weight, but most people never reach it. He asked me how I did it, and I told him my "secret"—diet and exercise! Just a few weeks later, in June 2009, I ran my first 5K at the age of forty-nine. Since then, I've done 8Ks, 10Ks, ten milers, and even a half-marathon!

I truly believe that as I get older, it is more important than ever to not only maintain my healthy eating and fitness habits but also to grow emotionally, to seek out new challenges and understanding. If I could share one piece of advice with other woman and men my age, it would be this: it is never too late to make changes to improve your physical and emotional health. And there is no better time to do it than right now.

Ten

FIND YOUR FITNESS

f you think you don't love exercise, you just haven't found the right exercise for *you*. So often, we force ourselves to engage in one type of exercise because we believe it's the "most effective." We'll grind our teeth through a thirty-minute session on the elliptical or spend more time dreading our run than actually running. I used to hate the stair climber with an intense and unrelenting passion, but I'd convince myself to do half an hour a few times a week because I thought it was such a good workout (which it is!). But then, one day I realized—what's the point in torturing myself? Exercise should be fun and uplifting.

Trust me—forcing yourself to do an activity that you don't feel passionate about is a surefire way to ensure you'll fall off the exercise bandwagon. Exercise is not one size fits all. The best type of exercise is the one that you *love* the most!

If you dread exercise, do an exercise experiment: commit to a different workout every week for two months. By trying eight different exercises, you're guaranteed to find something you enjoy.

While many people love the cardio machines and free weights of a typical gym experience, it's not right for everyone, and even the most devoted
gym rats can use a break every now and then. There are so many ways to
exercise. Mixing up your workouts and trying new activities is good for your
body and your mind. You'll tone different muscles in new ways and inject
a little variety into your routine. And—who knows?—you might even discover a new exercise passion.

Here are ten different ways to move your body:

Zumba

Zumba Basics: Fans describe Zumba as a "dance fitness party" and "exercise in disguise." Combining high-energy dance moves with aerobic elements, Zumba encourages participants to shimmy and shake and to samba,
salsa, merengue, and hip-hop. There are six different types of Zumba
classes—including classic Zumba, as well as classes for children and older
adults, pool-based classes, and classes that incorporate strength-training
elements—as well as a wide range of Zumba workout DVDs. Designed to
make fitness fun, the typical Zumba class lasts about an hour and includes
a warm-up, a variety of high-paced and slower songs, and a cooldown.

Zumba Benefits: The best thing about Zumba is that it's not just a
workout—it's an *experience*. Classes are notoriously upbeat, welcoming, and
friendly, and Zumba can be tailored to a variety of ages and fitness levels.
Many Zumba addicts came to their first class with little or no dance experience; newbies discover they can easily follow the rhythmic dance movements. But don't worry about hitting all the moves exactly as the instructor
demonstrates—Zumba is more about *feeling* the music with your body than
sticking to the perfect eight count. The upbeat Latin music energizes and
inspires, taking the pressure off to perform.

Zumba is a total-body workout that tones your legs, arms, and core while
improving cardiovascular fitness and coordination. Thanks to the aerobic

nature of the class, participants burn 350 to 700 (or more!) calories per class, depending on body size and intensity.

If you're starting from scratch, looking to make new friends, or searching for an energizing workout that doesn't really feel like a chore, Zumba might be the perfect fit.

Getting Started: Visit Zumba.com to find a class near you. Wear comfortable workout clothes that don't restrict your movements, and wear athletic shoes that you can pivot in. You'll also want to bring a bottle of water and a small towel to wipe away sweat.

ZUMBA INSIDER TIP

Diana, a Zumba instructor in Charlotte, North Carolina, admits that she was nervous about her first Zumba class. "When I first started doing Zumba, I worried about getting the moves right and if other people thought I was dancing weird. It was very stressful!" she says. "As I continued doing the class, I became more comfortable and finally decided to just let loose and focus on getting into the song and enjoying the moment, rather than doing a step properly or worrying what my neighbor thought. Once I let go, I really started to have fun and got an even better exercise!" Diana says the key is to dance like no one is watching.

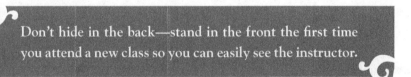

Don't hide in the back—stand in the front the first time you attend a new class so you can easily see the instructor.

Swimming

Swimming Basics: Most people already know how to doggy paddle around the pool, but swimming for fitness is a little different, focusing on swimming laps in a lane pool. In a pool set up for lap swimming, each lane is separated by a string of buoys and is usually 25 yards or 25 meters (known as short course) or 50 meters (long course) in length. There are many different strokes, but the front crawl/freestyle—face in the water; legs straight out behind you; and arms alternately raising overhead, in front, and then underwater toward the legs—is the most common.

Swimming Benefits: Water makes you feel nearly weightless, but it creates resistance. In many ways, swimming is the perfect exercise because it is a nonimpact form of aerobic exercise with built-in strength training; swimming is a gentle—but challenging—workout. Swimming works every major muscle group, including your legs, arms, core, rear, and back. It's a great alternative for people suffering from arthritis, chronic pain, fibromyalgia, joint conditions, and lower body injuries. Overweight individuals, whose joints are already stressed, may find that swimming is more comfortable than high-impact exercises because the water cushions the body through each movement.[42]

Even if swimming isn't your primary focus, it's an excellent form of cross-training because it builds your cardiovascular base and strengthens your muscles without inflicting impact on the joints, bones, and muscles.

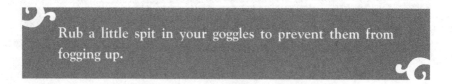

Rub a little spit in your goggles to prevent them from fogging up.

Getting Started: Swimming requires more than strength and endurance—it's a skill, too. Don't be frustrated if you don't get it right away. It will take several sessions to develop proper form and figure out how to balance each stroke with breathing. It's best to start off with small goals, such as swimming a length, resting for thirty seconds, and repeating ten times. Work slowly up to swimming longer durations and distances and supplement your swim workouts with other forms of cardio as you learn; it's unrealistic to expect that you'll pound out 2,000 meters in your first attempt.

Consider signing up for adult swim lessons or joining the U.S. Masters Swimming group at your pool. Don't be scared by the name—Masters simply means for adults and is open to all swimmers, regardless of skill or experience. Alternatively, you can watch swimming instructional videos on YouTube for easy-to-understand explanations of different strokes. At the pool, remember to follow basic pool etiquette. Share a lane with one other swimmer by sticking to one side, and share a lane with two other swimmers by circle-swimming (going up one side and back down the other; at most pools, circle swimming is conducted with each swimmer staying on the right side of the lane). Some pools will designate different lanes as fast, medium, or slow, and it's important to use the lane most appropriate for your ability.

In terms of equipment, at a minimum, you'll need a bathing suit, goggles, a swim cap, and access to a pool. Additional swimming equipment includes pull-buoys (flotation devices that rest between your thighs and isolate the effort in your upper body and help reinforce proper body alignment); kickboards (foam boards that isolate the effort in your lower body); fins (which strengthen your leg muscles); and hand paddles (which strengthen your arm muscles and improve stroke efficiency by emphasizing the power of different portions of the stroke). Some pools provide pull-buoys, kickboards, fins, and hand paddles to swimmers. If your pool doesn't have a pace clock, a waterproof watch allows you to time your splits (the duration between each length or lap).

Victoria, a swimmer and instructor from Washington, D.C., tells students to work on alignment before speed. "Ideally, while swimming freestyle, your body will be as close to horizontal as possible, with your hips at the surface and feet in line with your hips," she explains. "This is most easily accomplished by pressing down with your sternum to leverage the flotation provided by your lungs. At first, you will feel like you are swimming 'downhill,' but in the long run, you'll be much more efficient."

SWIM WORKOUT BASICS

You can always just hop in a pool and swim toward a certain distance goal, but swim workouts, with varying speeds and stroke types, will get you fitter, faster. Swim workouts read like a complex equation: "1 × 25? What's that? Ladder 500? Huh?" But once you know what the abbreviations and terms mean, it's actually pretty easy—and fun—to follow along a swim workout.

Swim workouts generally include a warm-up, main set, and cooldown. The main set will include repeat distances, sometimes simply called "repeats." When you see a "1 × 25," that means you swim 25 yards once; "5 × 100" means 100 yards, five times. The repeats may be followed by a specific time, such as "4 × 100 on 1:30"; this means you will swim 100 yards four times, starting every 1:30 minutes (the send-off interval). A workout may also specify that you should have a goal to hit a certain time, such as 1:20 for 100 yards; if a send-off interval is not specified, include a short break (10–30 seconds) in between each repeat distance. These sets might specify a certain stroke, such as breast, or piece of equipment, such as kick drills, which involve the kickboard.

Remember that times for a swim workout are always just suggestions; you should swim paces that work for you. A negative split swim involves swimming the second half of the specified distance faster than the first half. A descending set involves swimming each repeat faster than the one before it.

The most mentally stimulating swim workout may be the pyramid. Pyramids involve increasing and decreasing distances, with short rests in between. The main set below is an example of a pyramid workout. Remember—how many laps you'll swim depends on the size of your pool. Before you begin your first swim workout, ask an attendant about the pool length.

SAMPLE SWIM WORKOUT—1,000 METERS WITH PYRAMID

Warm-up: 1 × 200 easy meters

Main set: Pyramid with a 15-second rest in between each set.
Set includes: 1 × 50, 1 × 75, 1 × 100, 1 × 150, 1 × 100, 1 × 75 meters,
1 × 50 meters.

Cooldown: 1 × 200 easy meters

You can find more swim workouts at http://www.usms.org/training. A workout can be difficult to remember, so write it down on a piece of paper and stick it in a Ziploc bag. Leave the Ziploc on the pool edge at the end of your lane and double-check the details between sets.

Pilates

Pilates Basics: Pilates is a mat- and/or apparatus-based exercise routine that increases flexibility while building muscle strength. Pilates emphasizes the mind-body relationship and improves coordination. Although Pilates is a full-body workout, the exercises especially strengthen the core muscles, including the "corset" muscles: the abdominals and lower back.

The most common Pilates apparatus is the reformer, a gliding platform with a series of straps, pulleys, and springs. The springs create varying degrees of resistance while the user pushes and pulls from the platform; these movements are very precise and controlled. Pilates equipment also includes the magic circle, chair, barrel, and cadillac. Due to the price and size, most of this equipment is available only at Pilates studios. Pilates at your gym or on a DVD may be entirely mat-based and use body weight or resistance bands.

Pilates Benefits: The earliest adopters of Pilates were professional dancers—and for good reason! Pilates, which can be easily modified for all fitness levels, strengthens the core and creates long, lean muscles. The practice emphasizes fluid, strong movements instead of many repetitions of the same movement. By improving overall strength, Pilates improves posture, stabilizes the spine, and reduces or heals injuries.

The six principles of Pilates are concentration, control, centering, flow, precision, and breathing. Pilates isn't just a body exercise—it focuses on centering the mind and developing a sense of peace, too. Pilates enthusiasts say the mental and physical benefits of the practice carry over to the real world, too; they feel leaner, more graceful, and calmer.

Pilates is a low-impact exercise that strengthens and tones; however, it does not replace cardiovascular exercises. A well-rounded Pilates practice should be supplemented with several aerobic workouts, such as swimming or running, each week.

Getting Started: First-timers should start off with an introductory class at a specialized Pilates studio or gym. Classes allow newbies to receive immediate feedback from their certified Pilates instructor on their form; improper technique can lead to injury. Many studios suggest new students purchase private lessons for one-on-one attention.

Pilates can also be performed at home, using a Pilates DVD as a guide. At a minimum, you'll need a mat and comfortable clothing that you can bend and twist in. For less than thirty dollars, you can also purchase resistance bands or the Pilates magic circle.

SAMPLE PILATES MOVE: THE ROLL UP

Lie flat on your back, with your legs straight out in front of you and your arms reached out overhead. Inhale as you sweep your arms overhead and then toward your feet. Let your chin drop and your spine curl up. Exhale at the halfway point, using the release of breath to continue in an up-and-over movement, reaching your arms toward your toes. Use your breath and abdominal muscles, not the momentum from your arms, to pull your body forward. Keep your legs together, feet flexed, head tucked, and spine curved as you round up. Pause. Inhale as you slowly unfurl. Exhale when you are halfway, using your breath to guide you as you gently lower your back to the mat.

This move should be performed slowly and with controlled movements. Quality over quantity!

Trail Running

Trail Running Basics: Running down a city street inflicts a tremendous cognitive load on your brain—there's just so much information to process. Look at that building! Look at that man! Look at that sign! There's something to steal your attention everywhere you turn. Nature has the opposite effect; it calms, rejuvenates, and boosts mood.[43] Instead of sidewalks and treadmills, trail runners tackle hiking trails, rail-to-trails, and dirt paths. Trails vary in difficulty from dirt-packed paths in local parks to muddy mountain climbs.

Trail Running Benefits: Trail running, like road running, is an excellent cardiovascular exercise and lower-body strengthener. However, because trails are inherently less stable than the road, running on trails recruits additional muscles (especially in your core) to stabilize your body over the varying terrain. Trail running is a great option for runners who suffer from shin splints or minor joint pain, since trails are softer than roads, and every foot strike imparts less force on your body.

Trail running transports you away from the everyday stresses of modern life and into a more peaceful frame of mind. The natural scenery and challenging terrain command a different type of focus—while road runners may be tempted to zone out, trail runners often remark that the sport allows them to tune in.

> Every four to six weeks, "step back" your running by reducing overall mileage and intensity. This allows your body to heal and will ultimately make you a stronger, faster runner.

Getting Started: As with any exercise, it's important to ease into trail running. Let your body adjust by starting off on flat, dirt-packed, or gravel trails. If you're unfamiliar with the trails in your area, check out your city or state's parks and recreation department online. You can also ask a local running store for recommendations. Ease in with short walk/run sessions on the trail, and don't stress about time—you'll naturally be slower on softer trails than you are on the road or a treadmill.

While running on the trail, remember to keep your eyes on the ground, looking about five to eight feet in front of you so you can anticipate and react to obstacles. Take your time as you get used to stepping around rocks and sticks. Use your arms to balance yourself as you go up and down hills. And remember—safety must come first. Run with a buddy or carry a cell phone, and always let someone know where you're going and when you'll be back.

While you introduce yourself to the sport of trail running, you can wear normal running shoes. When you begin to run on the trails frequently or do longer distances, you may want to consider trail shoes. These shoes are more rigid, provide extra ankle support, and are designed to lock out more water and dirt than typical running shoes.

TRAIL ETIQUETTE

In order to protect the integrity of the natural environment, always run on designated trails. Leave nothing but sweat and footprints behind—don't litter.

If you approach another person on the trail, be sure to yell out, "On your left!" or "Good morning!" so you don't startle them as you pass. In general, the slower person should always yield to the faster person by stopping and moving to the side. Everyone should yield to horses.

Kettlebell

Kettlebell Basics: Ballistic training is a form of strength training that involves lifting, accelerating, and releasing weights such as the kettlebell. A kettlebell is a cast-iron weight that looks a little like a cannonball with a thick handle. The kettlebell's shape makes it an effective tool for ballistic training; the weight of the kettlebell is several inches below the handle, which makes it more difficult to control during movement. Combined with dynamic exercises, kettlebells will challenge and shape your body in entirely different ways than the traditional dumbbell because the kettlebell is lifted through a wider range of motion.

Kettlebell Benefits: Like traditional dumbbells, kettlebells come in a variety of weights, beginning at five pounds. Handling kettlebells builds muscle (especially in the core, legs, and shoulders); increases endurance; and strengthens grip. Perhaps the most notable benefits of working with kettlebells is that lifting one closely simulates real-world movements—for example, picking up a toddler and swinging him onto your hip.

While high-intensity kettlebell does provide a cardiovascular workout, you'll want to supplement your kettlebell routine with an aerobic activity, such as jogging or swimming.

Getting Started: Many gyms provide kettlebells and offer kettlebell group classes. Since kettlebell is so dynamic, it's important to perform the movements with the correct form. A session with a personal trainer who is familiar with kettlebell routines will help correct any issues and reduce the risk of injury.

Beginners should start off with a ten- or fifteen-pound kettlebell, which can be purchased online or in a fitness store. There are many kettlebell DVDs on the market, making kettlebell a great strength-training option for people who don't have access to a gym, as well as for parents of young children and people who live in colder climates.

YOUTUBE IT

If you're searching for kettlebell moves or other strength-training exercises, check out the online video site YouTube.com. Search for step-by-step videos created by personal trainers or other fitness professionals to ensure you use proper form.

Pole Dancing

Pole-Dancing Basics: In a low-lit room, ten women grasp shining silver poles and shimmy up and down. A scene from a gentlemen's club? Nope— it's just a pole-dancing fitness class. While critics may say the newest exercise craze glamorizes stripping, fans insist that it helps build muscle while boosting confidence. At a pole-dancing class, participants dance to energetic tunes and use the pole to increase strength, endurance, and flexibility.

Pole dancing is an excellent form of strength training—after all, you're hauling your entire body up and down the pole! Instructors often integrate abdominal work and dance sequences to provide a more total-body workout. You'll feel the workout in your arms, back, shoulders, chest, core, and rear.

Pole-Dancing Benefits: In addition to the physical benefits, pole-dancing fans say that the exercise increases self-esteem and body acceptance. Women—and men—of all sizes and shapes attend pole-dancing classes, which are not overly sexual but are fun and playful. If you're looking for a way to spice up your fitness, pole-dancing classes might be the hot ticket.

Getting Started: Pole-dancing fitness classes have become so popular that most urban areas boast at least one specialized studio. Classes are usually an hour in length. Seek out a beginner's class and introduce yourself to the instructor; she'll provide you with some quick tips on how to grasp and spin around the pole.

POLE-DANCING INSIDER TIP

"I love pole dancing because it makes me feel strong, sexy, and athletic. I don't do it for anyone else except myself," says Ceri, a twenty-four-year-old pole-dancing aficionado from Australia. "It's such an intense workout; I only need to do a couple classes a week to see serious results." Ceri recommends that first-timers wear shorts and a sleeveless top. "Your shorts don't need to be hot pants, but you need to be able to grip the pole with your thighs," she notes. And this is one workout you can actually do in high heels—"Heels always make classes more fun and help tone the legs and butt!" Ceri says. "But if you're attending a class for the first time and feel unsure, feel free to go barefoot."

BodyPump

BodyPump Basics: If you struggle to stick with a strength-training routine, BodyPump is a great alternative to lifting weights all alone. BodyPump is a group fitness class that incorporates the use of a weighted barbell, adjustable weighted plates, and an aerobic step. The high-intensity class, which is an hour long, is formatted around ten separate tracks set to energizing music. BodyPump starts and ends with a warm-up and a cooldown, and the eight tracks in between target a different muscle group—legs, chest, back, triceps, biceps, shoulders, and abdominals. During each track, the instructor will demonstrate strength-building moves—lunges, triceps extensions, dead rows, and overhead presses—using the barbell, plates, and step. The instructor may suggest weights for each track, but participants are urged to use weights that they are comfortable lifting.

BodyPump classes are highly standardized, so if you attend a class at one gym, it will be very similar to a class at another gym across town. But every three months, a new BodyPump class with fresh music and choreography is released, so classes never get stale.

BodyPump Benefits: Strength training is extremely important, especially for women, because it decreases body fat, develops strong bones, increases endurance, and reduces the risk of injury. It's easy to cut corners with strength training, but BodyPump encourages you to stick with it for an entire hour. In addition to working every major muscle group, lifting weights in such high, frequent repetitions means that BodyPump is also a calorie-blasting cardiovascular workout.

Getting Started: Seek out a BodyPump class at a local gym. Arrive fifteen minutes early and meet with the instructor. You'll need a weighted barbell, weighted plates, and an aerobic step. The instructor can help you figure out what weights to use. Since you'll be lifting many repetitions, it's wise to start off with lighter weights. Don't retreat to the back of the room—set up your step and weights near the front, where you can see the instructor.

BODYPUMP INSIDER TIP

Jen, a BodyPump instructor from Charlotte, North Carolina, says it's important to master proper weight-lifting form. "During your first few BodyPump classes, use a lighter weight and just focus on form and technique for all the exercises," she says. "Once you know how to safely execute the moves, you can increase your weight." For optimal results, Jen recommends attending two or three BodyPump classes each week.

Collect sample workouts from fitness magazines and stash them in a folder. Whenever you feel stuck in a rut, pull out a sheet at random.

Spinning

Spinning Basics: Cycling outside is fun, but it's dependent on so many factors. Snowing? Can't ride. Scary traffic? Don't want to ride! Spinning is a perfect alternative; if you love to cycle, you'll love spin class, a group class that utilizes specialized stationary upright bicycles. Each bike has a knob that can be adjusted with a simple flick of the wrist. Turning the knob one way will make the ride seem easier; turning the knob the other way will increase resistance and make the ride seem harder.

Throughout the one-hour class, the instructor will call out directions like, "Increase resistance by one turn!" or "Decrease resistance by two turns and pedal faster!" The pace often corresponds to the class's music; the instructor will tell everyone to "climb" a hill at a high resistance during a slow song or do sprints during an upbeat tune. Alternatively, the instructor might set a "relative scale," such as one through ten, with five being a challenging but doable resistance level for you. This way, she can say, "Turn it up to a seven!" and everyone can feel equally challenged but at different resistances. In addition to changing the resistance and pedal speed (known as cadence), you may spin in a variety of positions, such as standing up or hovering low over the seat. Ask the instructor to explain the positions to you before class starts.

Spinning Benefits: Spinning is many exercises in one: it provides an aerobic workout, increases muscle tone (especially in the legs), and boosts endurance. It is also a low-impact exercise, so it's easy on your joints. A great spin instructor will use music, words, and visualizations to help motivate you to push through your preconceived limits. It's an excellent class for a newbie exerciser, since you can make spin as easy (or hard!) as you want, thanks to the adjustable knob.

Getting Started: Spin classes are offered at many larger gyms. Arrive ten minutes before your first class, and ask the instructor to help adjust the seat and handlebar height to your body size. Correct settings are very important, since riding in the wrong position can cause pain and injury.

Spin bikes include cages on the pedals, so you can wear normal athletic shoes without your feet slipping; if you really enjoy spinning, there are clip-in shoes that allow more control over each pedal stroke. You'll want to invest in padded bike shorts, too, to help minimize soreness in your nether region.

GOING AT YOUR OWN PACE

Many people shy away from group fitness classes like spinning because they're afraid they won't be able to handle it. It's completely normal and acceptable to stop doing the exercise if you need a break; don't be embarrassed or ashamed. Everyone needs a breather every now and then. It's even okay to leave the room if you want fresh air. Just take the break in a discreet way so you don't interrupt others.

The only exception to this rule is during the final pose in a yoga class. Savasana, the corpse pose, requires that you lie perfectly still and empty your mind of any distracting thoughts. It's hard to feel Zen when someone is rolling up their yoga mat and stomping out of the room. So if you need to leave yoga early, do it before the final resting pose.

Interval Training

Interval Training Basics: Slow and steady may win the proverbial race, but fast and short can transform your workouts. Interval training can be applied to nearly any type of aerobic exercise—running, biking, swimming, or even dancing. Each interval consists of a burst of intense speed followed by a period of recovery, which means reduced speed but not stopping completely. The burst of speed should be performed at near-maximum exertion, while the recovery period should be much more comfortable.

Interval workouts can be performed on the track, the treadmill, the sidewalk, the elliptical machine, the stair climber, or even a spin bike; you can also do these workouts in a pool. Intervals, which are also called speedwork, may be measured by time or distance. You should always begin intervals with a minimum of a five-minute warm-up and a five-minute cooldown.

When using exercise equipment like an elliptical or a stair climber, vary the speed and resistance for a more effective workout.

Interval Training Benefits: Interval training is efficient and effective. You'll burn more calories—and build your endurance more quickly—in less time by doing interval workouts. The practice improves your cardiovascular capacity and trains your body to adjust to varying speeds. Furthermore, many research studies have found that interval training increases overall metabolism and triggers faster fat loss.[44]

Be careful—every workout shouldn't be an interval session. No matter what your sport, intervals are very hard on the body; it's wise to limit your interval training to one workout a week.

Getting Started: Start off by working four or five intervals into your next cardio session. For example, if you're planning to do a thirty-minute walk, do four intervals in the middle of your workout. Run for forty-five seconds, walk for forty-five seconds, and repeat three more times. Over time, you can increase the duration, intensity, and frequency of your intervals.

If you're basing intervals on time, you'll need to use a stopwatch, the timer on the exercise equipment, or a pace clock. You can base your intervals on distance if you're running around a track or using exercise equipment.

SAMPLE WALK/RUN INTERVAL WORKOUTS

Remember, "high intensity" means different things to different people—listen to your body!

LADDER INTERVAL (TOTAL DURATION: 14 MINUTES)
Start: 5-minute warm-up at low intensity
Interval 1: 15-second high intensity followed by a 15-second recovery at a moderate intensity
Interval 2: 30-second high intensity followed by a 30-second recovery
Interval 3: 45-second high intensity followed by a 45-second recovery
Interval 4: 1-minute high intensity followed by a 1-minute recovery
Finish: 5-minute cooldown at low intensity

1:1 INTERVAL (TOTAL DURATION: 18–30 MINUTES)
Start: 5-minute warm-up at low intensity
Interval: 1-minute high intensity followed by a 1-minute recovery at
  a moderate intensity
Repeat intervals 4–10 times
Finish: 5-minute cooldown at low intensity

CAMEL HUMPS INTERVAL (TOTAL DURATION: 24:15 MINUTES)
Start: 5-minute warm-up at low intensity
Interval 1: 15-second high intensity followed by a 30-second recovery at
  a moderate intensity
Interval 2: 30-second high intensity followed by a 30-second recovery
Interval 3: 45-second high intensity followed by a 30-second recovery
Interval 4: 1-minute high intensity followed by a 30-second recovery
Interval 5: 45-second high intensity followed by a 30-second recovery
Interval 6: 30-second high intensity followed by a 30-second recovery
Interval 7: 15-second high intensity followed by a 30-second recovery
Interval 8: 30-second high intensity followed by a 30-second recovery
Interval 9: 45-second high intensity followed by a 30-second recovery
Interval 10: 1-minute high intensity followed by a 30-second recovery
Interval 11: 45-second high intensity followed by a 30-second recovery
Interval 12: 30-second high intensity followed by a 30-second recovery
Interval 13: 15-second high intensity followed by a 30-second recovery
Finish: 5-minute cooldown at low intensity

Yoga

Yoga Basics: The translation of the word "yoga" is "to unite," and that's exactly what this calming exercise does—it unites your body, mind, and spirit. Spanning thousands of years, yoga is traditionally a mental practice that encourages spiritual introspection through meditation.

In modern times, yoga focuses more on the mind-body relationship, allowing yoga lovers (known as yogis) to reach inner peace through physical poses. Yoga is often simplified as a "stretching class," but it's so much more than that. Each pose is about creating strength, flexibility, and balance in the physical body and the mind. Yes, yoga is an exercise, but yogis get much more out of their practice than a physical workout. Many people return to yoga again and again because it provides them with a sense of peace and acceptance.

There are many different types of yoga. Although the poses are always the same, the types are very different (and vary further according to the studio and instructor). Classes are generally an hour to an hour and a half. The following are descriptions of the five most common styles taught in yoga studios across America.

- **Ashtanga:** A strenuous, fast-paced class that follows a standardized pattern of six series of pose sequences. An ashtanga class is challenging and requires a solid knowledge of a variety of poses. Yogis flow from one pose to the next quickly, in accordance with their breathing. At a Mysore ashtanga class, students will practice at their own pace in silence, without the instructor calling out poses.
- **Bikram:** Like ashtanga, Bikram is a challenging and advanced yoga. Bikram is performed in a hot, humid room—more than 100 degrees. The room is heated to encourage deeper breathing and muscle relaxation. Bikram also follows a standardized pattern of posing; Bikram yogis perform two cycles of twenty-six poses and two breathing exercises.
- **Hatha:** If you're a beginner, hatha yoga may be the perfect fit for you. Hatha classes are slower and typically offer more feedback from the instructor. Instead of quickly flowing from one pose to the next, hatha encourages yogis to focus on their breathing and positioning.
- **Power/Vinyasa/Flow:** Power yoga is a general term to describe an aerobic, very Westernized approach to the practice. Power yoga flows

quickly between poses, and there is an emphasis on breathing with movement. While an introductory power class would be fine for beginners, new students might feel lost in a fast-paced intermediate class. Many studios use the terms "power," "vinyasa," and "flow" interchangeably.

- **Prenatal**: Prenatal yoga classes are designed especially for pregnant women. Poses are modified to accommodate for the babies, and there's a heavier focus on breathing, stretching, and relaxing. Prenatal classes are also a great way to meet other expectant moms.

Additionally, many yogis choose to practice at home. You do not need an instructor to do yoga; you can practice in your living room, bedroom, backyard, hotel room, or even in the middle of a public park.

> Fold your yoga mat in half and then roll it up; this keeps the germy "outside" of the mat from touching the "inside."

Yoga Benefits: Yoga stretches muscles, boosts flexibility, and increases ranges of motion in the joints. The more aerobic styles boost endurance, improve cardiovascular health, and build muscle. All styles help create stronger core muscles, which improves posture. Many studies show that regularly practicing yoga can actually slow the heart rate and decrease blood pressure.

Breath is very important in yoga. One yogic breathing technique, known as ujjayi, has been shown to improve lung capacity and increase oxygenation. Ujjayi involves breathing air slowly through the nose with a slight constriction in the throat, filling the lungs deeply and completely, and exhaling slowly through the nose. A room of yogis engaging in ujjayi breathing sounds like ocean waves.

In addition to the physical benefits, yoga has been scientifically shown to boost mood, ease depression and anxiety, and reduce stress.

Getting Started: The easiest way to get started with yoga is to sign up for an introductory class at your gym or a local studio. Call ahead and ask which class would be best for beginners if you're not sure. You'll want to wear loose, comfortable clothing; most people are more comfortable in pants than shorts. Bring a yoga mat, a bottle of water, and a small towel. For hot yoga classes, bring a regular-size towel to lay on top of your yoga mat; you'll need it to absorb the sweat!

Before attending, do a little homework—look up the basic yoga positions. There are so many poses that it can feel overwhelming, and entering your first class with a vague idea of what's what will help greatly. Search the Internet for instructions on how to do the downward-facing dog, cobra, upward-facing dog, cat and cow, plank, warrior I and II, mountain, standing forward fold, chaturanga, child's pose, and corpse pose. And don't forget— you can always just look around to see what to do! Even experienced yogis do this when they are asked to do an unfamiliar pose.

As with any exercise class, introduce yourself to the instructor and mention that you're new to yoga; you'll get one-on-one attention to ensure you're doing the poses correctly. The instructor may offer you a block or strap; these tools are used to assist and support the body during challenging poses.

As mentioned, you don't need to go to a studio to practice yoga. You can buy yoga DVDs or download yoga podcasts and practice at home. Check out YogaJournal.com for tips.

DON'T COMPARE

Yoga is a judgment-free zone. In every class—introductory or advanced—you'll find yogis of all shapes and sizes. Some yogis can touch their toes; some cannot. Some yogis know every pose; some do not. It's important not to compare yourself to other people during a yoga class (and, heck, throughout life!). There is no "perfect" way to do a pose; the perfect execution is whatever you can do *today*.

Healthy Tipping Point Success Story: Kayla, 25, Canada

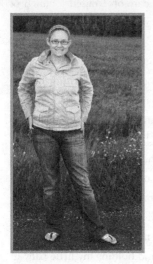

After months of trying for a baby, I got pregnant. My husband and I were nervous and ecstatic. Then, a few days shy of that magical twenty-week mark, my water broke. I was rushed to the hospital in an ambulance, and I could still feel my baby kicking away. I suppose that in the back of my mind I knew that not all pregnancies go as planned, but I was so far into the second trimester that I didn't think a miscarriage could possibly happen to me. Afterward, I experienced some of the darkest days of my life. I felt so much guilt that I wasn't able to carry James David to term. I felt I had failed myself and my husband.

Several months passed, and my husband and I were ready to try again. We were lucky and got pregnant after only two months. This time, we made it to twenty-three weeks, and then I started bleeding. I remember saying to my husband, "I just can't do this. I can't do this again."

I was airlifted to a regional hospital, where I was given drugs to try to slow down the delivery. My little girl was born early the next morning. She was tiny—only 500 grams—but she had a strong heartbeat and was able to breathe on her own. We named her Grace Johanna. Grace lived for two days. She suffered a major stroke during her second night. We held her as she passed away.

After we lost our two babies in the span of eight months, I could not just leap into another pregnancy. The idea just seemed overwhelming. And my self-image suffered so much after my two pregnancies. It made me so angry to look at my body, with its large stomach and extra weight, knowing that most people who are trying to lose pregnancy weight at least have a baby. I had the extra pounds and no baby to show for it. As a means of calming my anger and my sadness, I embraced running again. I had to start slow, following the couch-to-5K plan. I found a run on Mother's Day that was in support of the neonatal ICU where Grace was taken care of. I raised a bunch of money, trained really hard, and solidly ran the 5K three months after Grace was born.

I love the structure and commitment that training for a race provides. I felt like I needed to prove to myself that I could plan something and my body could cooperate with me and make it happen. So, I signed up for a half-marathon. I'm only six weeks into my training, but I love the physical and mental results that I am seeing from my half-marathon training. My body feels strong and fit. It is still not the same shape as it was before my pregnancies, but it has carried me 6.2 miles so far, and I look forward to training it to get me through 13.1 miles. This time—this training—is for me. It's a time to focus on my physical fitness and emotional recovery. These races are something I need to do. I run to heal my heart.

I look forward to getting pregnant again, and holding my little baby in my arms. No matter what, I will always carry my first two children in my heart. Once I finish my half-marathon, we've decided that we will try again to start our family.

Eleven

YOU (YES, YOU!) CAN RACE

There's something magical about crossing your first finish line. It's a mixture of excitement, relief, joy, and, of course, a little bit of exhaustion, too. Whether you dash to the end of a 5K, trudge through a triathlon, or walk/run a marathon, training for and completing in a race is a test of physical and mental endurance and strength. No matter how slow or fast, crossing a finish line will change the way you look at exercise—and yourself—forever.

Let's clear up something right away: "racing" isn't synonymous with "winning." Very few of us are destined to become Olympic athletes; if we're not having fun racing, what's the point? Racing doesn't imply that you are speedy or don't take walking breaks! Racing is about committing to a challenge, having fun, and testing your perceived limits. Racing is about discovering the depths of your physical and mental strength. Above all else, racing is simply about *experiencing*.

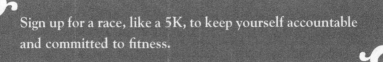

Sign up for a race, like a 5K, to keep yourself accountable and committed to fitness.

No matter what your fitness level, you can train to finish a race. Many newbies begin by doing a 5K (3.1 mile race). If you're starting from couch-potato scratch, a 5K will require about two months of training. Over time, you can work your way up to longer races, such as a 10K (6.2 miles) or even a full marathon. People of all shapes, sizes, and ages do races. Don't feel like you're too old, young, overweight, out-of-shape, or inexperienced to race. At a starting line, you'll see everybody from grandmas to teenagers to muscular running machines to pregnant ladies. More than 507,000 people finished a marathon in 2010, of which 41 percent were women and 35 percent were more than forty-five years old.[45]

The very best thing about signing up for a race is that *you are committed.* Racing is a great way to get and stay motivated to exercise. There's something about typing in your credit card number as you pay the entry fee! If you thrive under deadlines, you'll thrive in training. Sure, you can miss a training day here and there, but in general, if you want to feel prepared and do well, you need to stick to your schedule. Normally, adults don't have any deadlines for fitness; exercise is just something we're expected to do regularly, like brushing our teeth or unloading the dishwasher. But when you sign up for a race, you're challenging yourself: "In two months' time, I will run a 5K. I better get ready!"

COMMON RACE DISTANCES

5K = 3.1 miles

10K = 6.2 miles

15K = 9.3 miles

Half-Marathon = 13.1 miles

Marathon = 26.2 miles

Ultramarathon = Any distance beyond a marathon

Sprint Triathlon = Varies, but typically a 750-meter swim, a 12.5-mile
   bike, and a 5K run

Olympic/International Triathlon = Varies, but typically a 1,500-meter swim, a 24-mile bike, and a 10K run

Half Ironman = 1.2-mile swim, 56-mile bike, and a half-marathon

Ironman = 2.4-mile swim, 112-mile bike, and a marathon

Duathlon = A run, bike, and run of varying distances

Aquathon = A swim and a run of varying distances

Aquabike = A swim and a bike of varying distances

Metric = A 100K (62-mile) bike

Century = A 100-mile bike

Choose Wisely

Imagine running a race with 20,000 other people. Cheering spectators urge you up a challenging hill, there's a well-stocked water station every mile, a huge party awaits you at the finish line, and corporate sponsors lavish you with a well-stocked goodie bag. Now imagine running a race with 200 other people. It's peaceful and quiet, there's no bottle-necking at the start line, spectators are few and far between, and the lines for the bathroom aren't fifteen runners deep.

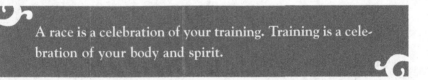

A race is a celebration of your training. Training is a celebration of your body and spirit.

All races aren't created equal. It's not that big races are always better than small races (or vice versa)—they're just *different*. And different types of races appeal to different people.

When it comes to selecting your first (or next) race, the first thing to consider, of course, is the race distance. There are people who select a long race—like a marathon—for their first race, but training for a race of this magnitude can feel overwhelming if it's your first time around the block. If you're new to running, a 5K or 10K would be an ideal first race. You can use these shorter distances as milestone markers for a longer race in the future, integrating the 5K or 10K training into your training plan for a longer race. You'll also want to consider the race's terrain; in addition to road races, there are trail races (for more information about trail running, check out page 283). While the training plan for a road race and a trail race are the same, it's wise to train on a trail at least once a week if you plan to compete in a trail race, since this allows your body to adjust to the terrain.

TIME IT RIGHT

To determine how long you'll need to train, check out the sample training plans that are provided in the next chapter. A 5K requires eight weeks of training; even with a solid fitness base, it will take at least twenty weeks to train for a marathon.

Additionally, you'll want to consider how any extra commitments and responsibilities will impact your ability to train. If you're very busy at work, it might not be the best time to do a half-marathon. If you hate to run outside in the snow, a midwinter 10K might not be ideal. Remember, never set yourself up to fail.

Once you've decided on your race criteria, search online or ask at a local running shop for race recommendations. Web sites such as Active.com and RunningRoom.com provide extensive lists of upcoming races across America and Canada.

You'll want to consider several additional factors beyond distance and timing: Do you want to run in a small race, which is usually cheaper but less showy, or a big race, which is more expensive but offers more amenities?

Are you willing to travel? Traveling for races can be fun, but remember to factor in the cost of transportation, hotel, food, and time off from work. What is the course like? Is it flat, shaded, or hilly? Check the race's Web site for a course description or an elevation profile to determine whether the race is easy, moderate, or challenging. Last, what is the race's time limit? This is especially important if you're planning on using a walk/run method, as described below, or are tackling an endurance event for the first time. Some races are more accommodating to walkers than others; large city races may impose strict time limits on racers because they need to reopen the streets to car traffic as soon as possible.

When you find your ideal race, sign up! Pay that race entry fee. You'll get a discount for registering early and monetarily committing to the race will be a motivating kick in the running shorts.

Train Smart

Most people do too much, too hard, and too soon. More isn't always better. In fact, sometimes more is the exact opposite of what you need. Your body requires time to adjust to the rigors of training. Over time, training strengthens your bones, stabilizes your joints, and increases muscle mass so that you can handle longer distances and greater effort. If you jump ahead too fast, you're setting yourself up for injury—a strained muscle, a bone stress fracture, or mental burnout could result. Whatever the distance, it's a smart idea to use a training plan.

HEALTHY TIPPING POINT
TRAINING PLANS

Training plans for a variety of race distances are provided in Chapter 12.

Walk Your Way to Success

It's okay to walk. Actually, it's more than okay to walk—taking walk breaks is safe, healthy, motivating, and can actually improve your overall time. Let's say it takes you twelve minutes to jog a mile. If you scheduled regular walk breaks—say, a forty-five-second walk for every two minutes of running—your average pace per mile may drop. By walking, you'll feel more refreshed during the run intervals and actually cover the distance more quickly than you would've otherwise. And taking a walk break doesn't mean you aren't a real runner! So instead of fighting the urge to walk, take *purposeful* walking breaks.

- **Walk/Run Intervals:** If you're a running newbie, using a walk/run interval, as described below, can help you build endurance. Some runners use a 1:1 ratio, others run for four minutes and walk for thirty seconds. Experiment a bit with your workouts to discover what works for you. Over the course of several weeks, you can decrease the amount of time you spend walking and transition to running more frequently.

- **Walk Before the Going Gets Tough:** Don't wait to walk until you're absolutely exhausted; take a short break *before* the point of no return. You won't feel as depleted and will find it easier to start back up again.

- **Use Visual Cues:** If you're not following a timed interval schedule but need a walking break, use a landmark to determine when you'll begin running again. Select a tree or street sign in the distance and tell yourself, "When I get to that spot, I will begin to run again." When you're about five feet away from the landmark, pick up your pace and pat yourself on the back for speeding up early (a silly motivational trick that really works!).

- **Walk Smart:** If it's very hot out, time your walks so you're in the shade. If you're running a hilly course, walk up hills to give your legs a break. If you have knee troubles, it may be wise to walk down steep hills as well.

- **Suitable for All Distances:** The walk/run philosophy can be applied to any training plan and any race distance. Many people walk/run 5Ks; many people walk/run marathons.

"CAN I TRAIN ENTIRELY ON THE TREADMILL?"

Training isn't just about increasing endurance, muscular strength, and cardiovascular fitness; it's also about preparing your body for the rigors of the final race distance. It's important to train at least partially on the appropriate terrain, such as sidewalks for a road race or trails for a trail race. A treadmill provides significantly more give than a slab of concrete. While it certainly is possible to train for a shorter distance on a treadmill, you'll risk injuring yourself on the day of the race, since your body will not be used to the shock of pounding the pavement.

Another factor to consider is that the treadmill's belt pushes you slightly forward, making the run feel a little easier than it would if you were running outside. One way to compensate for this effect is to always set the incline on a treadmill to at least 1.5–2.0 percent grade. You'll also want to run "hills" on the treadmill, occasionally pushing the grade up to 5 percent or higher to simulate outdoor settings.

If you're used to running on the treadmill and want to move outdoors, transition slowly in order to allow your body time to adjust. Begin by doing one short run outside each week, gradually increasing the frequency and distance of outdoor runs over several weeks.

MAKING YOUR PLAN WORK FOR YOU

There isn't one way to train for a race. Everyone's body, schedule, and goals are different. Some people can handle running a high mileage each week; others cannot run short distances more frequently than three times a week without risking injury. It's important to consider that training plans are designed to get the largest number of racers safely across the finish line; this doesn't mean all plans will work well for everyone. Don't feel forced to stick with a plan if you're feeling too sore, exhausted, sick, or just emotionally burned out.

> Training plans are guidelines, not absolutes. Listen to your body; don't blindly follow a plan.

You'll notice that the Healthy Tipping Point training plans, as well as other training plans available in other books and online, include rest days. Remember—more is not always better! Resting is an extremely important part of training for a race of any distance (and for exercise in general).

Rest days give your muscles time to repair. When you exercise, the muscles are stressed, which creates very small tears in the muscular tissue. The repair process utilizes protein from the foods you eat to strengthen your muscles. It sounds counterintuitive, but you must break down a muscle before you can repair it and build it stronger than before. If you don't give your body the rest it needs, your muscles will be in a constant state of breakdown with no repair period, and you may experience symptoms of overtraining, including constant pain, exhaustion, frequent or reoccurring injuries, headaches, emotional turmoil, and decreased performance.

When you see "rest" on your training plan, you have two options: you can take the day off entirely or swap in a *very* light workout. It's a good idea to completely skip all forms of exercise if you're feeling rather sore from your previous workouts or are training for a long event, like a half-marathon or a marathon. It's also wise to rest completely if you're feeling emotional burnout from training. If you must move on your rest day, engage in low-intensity exercise such as a short walk or a leisurely bike ride around the neighborhood.

You may discover that you need more rest days than your training plan suggests. If you feel extra tired or sore, take an additional rest day; there's a point at which the cost of exercise overrides the benefits.

Many new racers fly into a panic if they miss a scheduled workout. "I've got a meeting and cannot do this five miler!" they'll moan. "I'm totally screwed!" Remember that training plans are not absolutes. If you miss a scheduled workout, creating an accidental rest day, consider making up your workout on the next rest day. Before doing this, double-check that you won't tinker with the rhythm of rest days and force your body to work extra hard many days in a row. For example, if you miss a five-mile run, you won't want to try to make it up the day before your long run of the week, since your legs will feel incredibly fatigued during the longer run. If you miss your weekly long run, it's wise to eliminate another day of running and do the long run then.

In general, it's really not a big deal if you miss a workout—or even a few workouts—in your training plan. All training plans build in room for missed workouts. You don't want to make skipping workouts a habit, but don't get stressed out if life gets in the way every now and then. After all, this is about having fun, not smashing any world records! If you find yourself missing more and more days, review your race's Web site to see if you could drop down to a shorter distance (many half-marathons also offer a 5K or 10K).

When you see "cross-training" on your training plan, this means you should do an activity beyond your core exercise. Cross-training allows you to continue to build endurance and strength while giving your body a break. If you're training for a running race, choose a low- or no-impact form of cross-training, such as swimming, the elliptical, or cycling.

RUNNING BACK-TO-BACK DAYS

If you're constantly sore or struggling with lower-body injuries, eliminate back-to-back runs from your schedule. Many people find they cannot handle running two days in a row or more than four days a week. Slip a rest day or cross-training day in between your runs.

Last, but certainly not least, remember that a training plan is not only just a guideline, it's also not a firm schedule. A training plan doesn't know what days you have off from work. A training plan cannot predict when you're going to get the flu. A training plan doesn't account for your child puking through the night and keeping you up until dawn. Many training plans are formatted in a Monday through Sunday format, but you can play around with the schedule to make it work for you. For example, if you work a Saturday and Sunday shift, it might be easier to do your long run on a Tuesday. Before you make any switches, just be sure to study the pattern of workouts and rest days to ensure you don't shuffle too many hard workouts one right after the other.

GROSS-OUTS AND INJURIES

Signing up for a race and following a training plan will make you feel incredibly tough—because you truly are awesome for tackling such a challenge! As you trudge through weeks and weeks of training, you'll discover that racing isn't all glory; sweat, blisters, and snot rockets can be a little gross, too.

Don't tackle speed and distance goals at the same time. Too much, too soon is a recipe for a training disaster.

Unfortunately, training can also lead to painful injuries. The easiest way to prevent injuries from happening in the first place is to go very slowly. Any time you add something new to your workouts—higher mileage, running on a new surface, doing speedwork, running on hills—integrate it into your schedule over several weeks. An old running rule of thumb is not to increase your total mileage per week by more than 10 percent as you train for a race. For example, if you ran ten miles in the first week of training, run eleven miles total during the second week.

By training smart—and following a few simple tricks—you can keep your training as safe and fun as possible.

- **Chafing:** Chafing occurs when your skin rubs up against clothing or another body part. It looks and feels like a rug burn, but chafing can be incredibly painful, stopping you dead in your tracks in the middle of a workout. The most common chafing areas are in between the thighs, the armpits, under the breasts, along the sports bra line, and along the waist.

  To prevent chafing, you'll want to apply a slippery substance, like Body Glide (available online and at running specialty stores) or Vaseline, to the area before you begin your workout. If you find you sweat through these substances, try lining the chafe area with athletic tape, which will serve as a barrier. The best solution for thigh chafing is to wear longer, skintight spandex shorts or capris (you can wear them under looser shorts, if you want). Before buying athletic clothing, always inspect the seams for rough edges; these areas are the most likely to cause chafing.

- **Blisters:** Blisters are so small, and yet they can wreak so much havoc. To prevent them from occurring, rub Body Glide or Vaseline on your feet before putting on your socks. Moleskin, a thick padding available in the foot-care aisle at most pharmacies, can be applied over blister-prone spots like an extra-thick and super-sticky Band-Aid. If you get blisters on the bottom of your feet, try sweat-wicking, not cotton, socks. If you get blisters in between your toes, purchase running toe socks. Toe socks wrap each toe individually in sweat-wicking fabric. Last, consider switching shoes; if you get blisters in the same spot constantly, it can be a sign that your shoes don't fit properly.

• **Knee Pain:** Knee pain is a very common type of running injury, especially for new female runners. Many women have weak quadriceps and tight hamstrings, which causes the patellar bone (the kneecap) to track out of place through each stride. This tracking causes a condition known as patellofemoral pain syndrome, commonly referred to as runner's knee. Symptoms of runner's knee include pain behind or below the kneecap and pain, popping, or grinding sensations when you bend your knee, sit for long periods, or walk downstairs or downhill. Runner's knee can also be caused by running on a slope (for example, the side of a road) or running in improperly fitted or old shoes.

To cure runner's knee, take *at least* a week off from running and ice your knees several times a day for fifteen minutes at a time. When you begin to run again, step back the frequency and intensity of your running, take more walking breaks, stop at the first sign of pain, and ice your knees after every workout to prevent swelling. Icing is effective, but it's simply symptom management. You'll want to strengthen your quadriceps so your kneecap stays in position through your workouts. To build muscle, do two or three sets of five to ten thirty-second wall sits every day (squat against a wall with your knees at a 90-degree angle and your feet directly under your ankles). Additionally, consider meeting with a physical therapist to learn additional strength-building and stabilizing exercises.

Cross-training is another way to ward off knee pain, since you'll strengthen your leg muscles more evenly by doing different types of exercise. Swimming is the ideal type of cross-training for people who suffer from joint pain.

Not all knee pain is runner's knee, so if the pain continues or worsens, reach out to a sports medicine doctor. Call your local running store and ask the manager for a recommendation for a doctor who is well versed in running injuries.

- **Digestive Issues:** Don't be embarrassed—many racers suffer from "runner's trots." Running causes your intestines to jostle around and directs more blood toward your legs; this can trigger an uncontrollable urge to use the bathroom. Most runners find that they *must* use the bathroom before going on a run or they experience discomfort.

  If you continue to have problems, look at your fueling: you may not be able to eat a large or fiber-rich meal immediately before your run. Some people need more than an hour of digestion time before exercising. You might also want to experiment with avoiding soda, spicy foods, dairy, and over-the-counter painkillers like ibuprofen during the twenty-four hours before a run.

  So, what do you do if you have to *go* during a run? First, slow to a walk. If there is a supermarket, gas station, or restaurant nearby, pop into the bathroom. And yes—many runners (I'll admit it . . . like myself) have gone behind a bush and done their business in emergency situations. Consider it a badge of honor. When you've gotta go, you gotta go!

- **Other Aches and Pains:** Running is very high impact and can lead to lots of aches and pains. How do you know what is normal soreness and what's the beginning of an injury? One way to distinguish the two is that normal soreness is usually generalized ("My legs ache from that long run!") and an injury is specific and acute ("A spot right above my ankle is killing me!"). If the sensation is present during normal activities (such as walking upstairs), it may be an injury.

  If you even *suspect* you may have an exercise-induced injury, stop exercising immediately. Take off a few days—or even weeks or months—until you can slowly return to exercise and experience no pain. It can be disconcerting to take so much time off, especially if you're just beginning to experience your Healthy Tipping Point or are training for your first race, but it is necessary. You cannot heal an injury by exercising through it. You need to rest! If you maintain healthy eating habits, you will not undo all your hard work. You may also be able to do other exercises to maintain your endurance; again, try swimming or biking. If the pain is very acute or if you've taken several weeks off and there's been no improvement, consider making an appointment with a sports medicine doctor, since some injuries must be surgically repaired.

Setting Race Goals

Congratulations! You've made it through training, and now it's time to tackle your race. The race is a celebration of your training, and while it's natural to feel nervous, try to remember that you're out there to have fun.

One way to take the pressure off is to set realistic race goals. Many racers get caught up in hitting a certain finishing time (known as "PRs" or personal records). Time-based goals can drive you crazy and can lead to intense feelings of disappointment at the finish line. Set your goals based on other factors; if it's your first time running a particular distance, make it your goal to simply *finish*. You could also try to run more than you walk, maintain a positive attitude throughout the entire course, or have enough strength to sprint the last 300 yards. Your goals could also revolve around running a "smart" race; you could aim to run a negative split, when the second half of the race is faster than the first.

It's especially important to set your goals based on what you are capable of at the current time. Basing your goals on what your friends can do is pointless; you're *you*! Everyone's fitness ebbs and flows, so don't beat yourself up if you're not in the shape you were a year ago. Just focus on doing your personal best right now.

Part of what makes racing so much fun is that *anything* can happen; you never know how it's going to go until you're racing. Your performance hinges on many factors, including the course's elevation profile, the weather, and the crowd. If you do set a time goal, make sure it's flexible. Adjust your goals throughout your training and on race morning, if necessary. It's also helpful to set A, B, and C goals. Your A goal could be to simply finish; the B goal would be to run a moderately fast race; and your dream finishing time would be your C goal. No matter what, if you set multiple time- and nontime-based goals, you'll finish feeling proud and happy.

In the week before your race, review the race Web site for all the last-minute information you'll need, including where and when to pick up your race packet and where to park. Also review the course map; you may want to bring your own water if you feel there aren't enough water stations (which is more common for smaller races). The night before your race, check the weather forecast and lay out an appropriate outfit. Pin your bib number to your shirt and tie your timing chip to your shoe, if you have them already. Set out any food or gear you're planning to bring to the race so you don't forget anything at the last moment. Consider bringing a change of clothes for after the race.

TAPER

For longer races, training plans include a taper period, which is when you dial back the mileage and allow your body to rest in preparation for the big day. A marathon taper usually lasts two weeks, but a taper for a 10K might be only a few days. Tapering can be nerve-wracking, but trust your plan—the taper period is extremely important, and you'll feel fresh and prepared on race day!

It can be difficult to get a full night's sleep before a race, but don't worry—research shows it's just as important to sleep well in the days preceding the race. If you get anxious, envision a successful race. Then, get your mind off your race; try counting back from 300 by threes. I swear that this trick works—and it helped me conk out before my first marathon.

Remember the number two rule of racing: Never do anything new on race day. Don't wear anything new; don't eat anything new. Part of your training was figuring out what clothes and food you can count on. Switching it up at the last moment rarely ends well.

You may be wondering, "What's the number one rule of racing?" The most important thing to remember is to always have fun. You have worked so hard and experienced tremendous mental and physical strength. A few months ago, you might not have believed you were capable of finishing this race, but today, you will. You can do anything—enjoy the ride!

Healthy Tipping Point Success Story: Kristine, 39, Canada

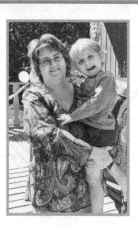 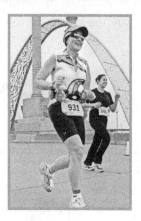

After two babies, a divorce, another marriage, and another baby, I put more weight on my already overweight frame. In January 2006, I was thirty-three years old and weighed 243 pounds. I had a great marriage, but the weight made me physically uncomfortable, I was miserable at work, we had financial problems, and I suffered from terrible anxiety.

For a long time, losing weight was all about getting skinny, so I tried so many different fad diets. Some were reasonably legit, many were trendy, many were expensive, and few or none addressed my issues of why I overate in the first place. On these diets, I would eventually plateau, quit, and regain the weight for one reason or another. I felt like a failure, which only encouraged me to continue to overeat.

My doctor, who had long been encouraging me to lose weight, prescribed an antidepressant to combat my anxiety and help me sleep. I began to diet and exercise, too, and I lost about thirty pounds. Coupled with a new job, my anxiety levels were under control.

One day, I heard about the Arthritis Foundation's Joints in Motion program; runners complete a half-marathon and fund-raise for the society. My mother suffers from terrible arthritis in the knee; the disease restricted her life—she couldn't go on walks or play golf, and she was taking painkillers every day. At thirty-five years old, I still had healthy limbs, and I wanted to do the race in her honor.

There were definitely days when my goal—13.1 miles—seemed so far away. I trained for months, mostly by myself because I wanted to run at my own pace. My husband, who was a total couch potato at the time, supported me but thought I was crazy (he's since transformed his life, too, and runs marathons—who's crazy now?).

Joints in Motion, which provided online coaching and training, was simply about finishing the half-marathon and raising money; time didn't matter. This really boosted my confidence! I finished the race in 3:21, which felt like a huge success. Since then, I've run six half-marathons and brought my finish time down to 2:03:57! Thanks to running and eating better, I've lost 107 pounds!

Focusing on completion, and not time, taught me that finishing really can be enough. And if you do have a goal time and miss it, there will always be another race. Not finishing or not hitting your goal time is not failing. Failing is not trying at all.

Twelve

HEALTHY TIPPING POINT TRAINING PLANS

Remember that training plans are just guidelines, not absolutes. Always consult with your doctor before beginning any exercise program. Here are some other things to keep in mind:

- Some plans call specifically for walk/run intervals. These intervals should be completed at paces that are comfortable for you.
- Some of the plans give distances but do not specify walk/run intervals; however, you can use the walk/run interval method to train for any race distance. You can use the interval method even if it's not on the plan. Never be afraid to walk!
- On days labeled "cross-train," do an alternative activity, such as yoga, Zumba, cycling, or swimming. Additionally, strength training will help ward off injuries.
- On days labeled "rest," set aside ten minutes for gentle stretching.
- On days labeled "speedwork," you'll complete several intervals of sprints at 90 percent performance. "3 × 400" signals 3 sets of 400-meter (roughly 0.25-mile) sprints. Take a thirty-second to one-minute walking or jogging break in between each sprint.

- Remember to always start and end by walking for two to five minutes as warm-up and cooldown; this is in addition to the time/distance suggested on the training plan.
- You should stretch before and after all workouts.
- If you are tired, unusually sore, or sick, don't feel pressured to do the workout just because it's on your plan. Rest!
- If you feel a nagging injury coming on, take *at least* a week off from running and then test it out with a very short, slow run. If the ache continues, stop running and see a doctor. If you experience any acute pain, stop running and see a doctor right away.
- If you miss a long run, do it later in the week (instead of a shorter run), if possible. Time it carefully; don't complete two long runs too close together.
- If a workout seems too difficult or you feel like the plan jumps ahead too quickly, step back and repeat the previous week or simply extend the walk intervals by fifteen to thirty seconds.

A Start-from-Scratch Walk/ Run 5K Training Plan

Even if you've never thought of yourself as a runner, you can train to complete a 5K in eight weeks. If the goal seems insurmountable now, trust me—it's definitely achievable! The secret is using a walk/run training plan, which allows you to slowly increase endurance and strength without ever feeling overwhelmed by the workouts. A walk/run training plan like the one below is based on time, not distance.

Monday	Tuesday	Wednesday	Thursday	Friday	Saturday	Sunday
WEEK 1						
Rest	Total: 20 minutes. For 10 minutes: Alternate jogging for 30 seconds and walking for 90 seconds. For 10 minutes: Walk briskly.	Rest	Cross-train	Total: 20 minutes. For 10 minutes: Alternate jogging for 30 seconds and walking for 90 seconds. For 10 minutes: Walk briskly.	Rest	Total: 25 minutes. For 15 minutes: Alternate jogging for 30 seconds and walking for 90 seconds. For 10 minutes: Walk briskly.
WEEK 2						
Rest	Total: 20 minutes. For 15 minutes: Alternate jogging for 45 seconds and walking for 60 seconds. For 5 minutes: Walk briskly.	Rest	Cross-train	Total: 25 minutes. For 20 minutes: Alternate jogging for 45 seconds and walking for 90 seconds. For 5 minutes: Walk briskly.	Rest	Total: 25 minutes. For 20 minutes: Alternate jogging for 45 seconds and walking for 60 seconds. For 5 minutes: Walk briskly.

Monday	Tuesday	Wednesday	Thursday	Friday	Saturday	Sunday
WEEK 3						
Rest	Total: 25 minutes. For 15 minutes: Alternate jogging for 45 seconds and walking for 45 seconds. For 10 minutes: Walk briskly.	Rest	Cross-train	Total: 30 minutes. For 20 minutes: Alternate jogging for 45 seconds and walking for 60 seconds. For 10 minutes: Walk briskly.	Rest	Total: 30 minutes. For 20 minutes: Alternate jogging for 45 seconds and walking for 45 seconds. For 10 minutes: Walk briskly.
WEEK 4						
Rest	Total: 25 minutes. For 20 minutes: Alternate jogging for 45 seconds and walking for 45 seconds. For 5 minutes: Walk briskly.	Rest	Cross-train	Total: 30 minutes. For 25 minutes: Alternate jogging for 45 seconds and walking for 60 seconds. For 5 minutes: Walk briskly.	Rest	Total: 30 minutes. For 25 minutes: Alternate jogging for 45 seconds and walking for 45 seconds. For 5 minutes: Walk briskly.

Monday	Tuesday	Wednesday	Thursday	Friday	Saturday	Sunday
WEEK 5						
Rest	Total: 25 minutes. For 20 minutes: Alternate jogging for 60 seconds and walking for 45 seconds. For 5 minutes: Walk briskly.	Rest	Cross-train	Total: 30 minutes. For 25 minutes: Alternate jogging for 60 seconds and walking for 60 seconds. For 5 minutes: Walk briskly.	Rest	Total: 30 minutes. For 25 minutes: Alternate jogging for 60 seconds and walking for 45 seconds. For 5 minutes: Walk briskly.
WEEK 6						
Rest	Total: 30 minutes. For 25 minutes: Alternate jogging for 60 seconds and walking for 45 seconds. For 5 minutes: Walk briskly.	Rest	Cross-train	Total: 35 minutes. For 30 minutes: Alternate jogging for 60 seconds and walking for 60 seconds. For 5 minutes: Walk briskly.	Rest	Total: 35 minutes. For 30 minutes: Alternate jogging for 60 seconds and walking for 45 seconds. For 5 minutes: Walk briskly.

Monday	Tuesday	Wednesday	Thursday	Friday	Saturday	Sunday
WEEK 7						
Rest	Total: 30 minutes. For 25 minutes: Alternate jogging for 60 seconds and walking for 30 seconds. For 5 minutes: Walk briskly.	Rest	Cross-train	Total: 35 minutes. For 30 minutes: Alternate jogging for 60 seconds and walking for 45 seconds. For 5 minutes: Walk briskly.	Rest	Total: 35 minutes. For 30 minutes: Alternate jogging for 60 seconds and walking for 30 seconds. For 5 minutes: Walk briskly.
WEEK 8						
Rest	Total: 35 minutes. For 30 minutes: Alternate jogging for 60 seconds and walking for 30 seconds. For 5 minutes: Walk briskly	Rest	Cross-train	Total: 20 minutes. For 15 minutes: Alternate jogging for 60 seconds and walking for 30 seconds. For 5 minutes: Walk briskly	Rest	5K Race

Owning the 5K Training Plan

If you can already walk/run for twenty-five minutes, this training plan will help you increase endurance and cross the 5K finish line faster than before.

Monday	Tuesday	Wednesday	Thursday	Friday	Saturday	Sunday
WEEK 1						
Rest	Speedwork: Jog for 5 minutes. 3 × 400 m / 1-minute walking or jogging break in between. Jog for 10 minutes.	Rest	Cross-train	Total: 25 minutes. For 20 minutes: Alternate jogging for 60 seconds and walking for 30 seconds. For 5 minutes: Walk briskly.	Rest	Run 1.5 miles with minimal walk breaks. For 5 minutes: Walk briskly.
WEEK 2						
Rest	Speedwork: Jog for 5 minutes. 4 × 400 m / 1-minute walking or jogging break in between. Jog for 10 minutes.	Rest	Cross-train	Total: 30 minutes. For 25 minutes: Alternate jogging for 60 seconds and walking for 30 seconds. For 5 minutes: Walk briskly.	Rest	Run 2 miles with minimal walk breaks. For 5 minutes: Walk briskly.

Monday	Tuesday	Wednesday	Thursday	Friday	Saturday	Sunday
WEEK 3						
Rest	Speedwork: Jog for 5 minutes. 4 × 400 m / 1-minute walking or jogging break in between. Jog for 10 minutes.	Rest	Cross-train	Total: 35 minutes. For 30 minutes: Alternate jogging for 60 seconds and walking for 30 seconds. For 5 minutes: Walk briskly.	Rest	Run 2 miles with minimal walk breaks. For 5 minutes: Walk briskly.
WEEK 4						
Rest	Speedwork: Jog for 10 minutes 4 × 400 m / 1-minute walking or jogging break in between. Jog for 10 minutes.	Rest	Cross-train	Total: 35 minutes. For 30 minutes: Alternate jogging for 60 seconds and walking for 30 seconds. For 5 minutes: Walk briskly.	Rest	Run 2.5 miles with minimal walk breaks. For 5 minutes: Walk briskly.

Monday	Tuesday	Wednesday	Thursday	Friday	Saturday	Sunday
WEEK 5						
Rest	Speedwork: Jog for 10 minutes 5 × 400 m / 1-minute walking or jogging break in between. Jog for 10 minutes.	Rest	Cross-train	Total: 35 minutes. For 30 minutes: Alternate jogging for 90 seconds and walking for 30 seconds. For 5 minutes: Walk briskly.	Rest	Run 2.5 miles with minimal walk breaks. For 5 minutes: Walk briskly.
WEEK 6						
Rest	Speedwork: Jog for 10 minutes 6 × 400 m / 1-minute walking or jogging break in between. Jog for 10 minutes.	Rest	Cross-train	Total: 40 minutes. For 35 minutes: Alternate jogging for 90 seconds and walking for 30 seconds. For 5 minutes: Walk briskly.	Rest	Run 3.0 miles with minimal walk breaks. For 5 minutes: Walk briskly.

Monday	Tuesday	Wednesday	Thursday	Friday	Saturday	Sunday
WEEK 7						
Rest	Speedwork: Jog for 10 minutes 6 × 400 m / 1-minute walking or jogging break in between. Jog for 10 minutes.	Rest	Cross-train	Total: 40 minutes. For 35 minutes: Alternate jogging for 90 seconds and walking for 30 seconds. For 5 minutes: Walk briskly.	Rest	Run 3.5 miles with minimal walk breaks. For 5 minutes: Walk briskly.
WEEK 8						
Rest	Run 2.0 miles without walking.	Rest	Cross-train	Total: 25 minutes. For 20 minutes: Alternate jogging for 90 seconds and walking for 30 seconds. For 5 minutes: Walk briskly.	Rest	5K Race!

Your First 10K Training Plan

Before starting this plan, you should be able to run three miles with minimal walking breaks. You also should be running at least nine miles per week and have a minimum of two months of running experience under your belt. If you're just getting started, begin with the Start-from-Scratch Walk/Run 5K Training Plan and/or Owning the 5K Training Plan.

Walk/run intervals are not specifically labeled in this plan. However, you can use the walk/run interval method to train for a 10K.

Week Five of this plan is a step-back week, which is when you reduce mileage to give your body and mind a break.

Monday	Tuesday	Wednesday	Thursday	Friday	Saturday	Sunday
WEEK 1						
Cross-train or rest	Speedwork: Run for 10 minutes 4 × 400 m / 30-second walking or jogging break in between. Run for 10 minutes.	Rest	Cross-train	2.5 miles	Rest	3.0 miles
WEEK 2						
Cross-train or rest	Speedwork: Run for 10 minutes 4 × 400 m / 30-second walking or jogging break in between. Run for 15 minutes.	Rest	Cross-train	3.0 miles	Rest	3.5 miles

Monday	Tuesday	Wednesday	Thursday	Friday	Saturday	Sunday
WEEK 3						
Cross-train or rest	Speedwork: Run for 10 minutes 5 × 400 m / 30-second walking or jogging break in between. Run for 15 minutes.	Rest	Cross-train	3.5 miles	Rest	4.0 miles
WEEK 4						
Cross-train or rest	Speedwork: Run for 10 minutes 5 × 400 m / 30-second walking or jogging break in between. Run for 15 minutes.	Rest	Cross-train	3.5 miles	Rest	4.5 miles
WEEK 5						
Cross-train or rest	3.0 miles	Rest	Cross-train	3.0 miles	Rest	3.0 miles
WEEK 6						
Cross-train or rest	Speedwork: Run for 10 minutes 5 × 400 m / 30-second walking or jogging break in between. Run for 15 minutes.	Rest	Cross-train	3.5 miles	Rest	5.0 miles

Monday	Tuesday	Wednesday	Thursday	Friday	Saturday	Sunday
WEEK 7						
Cross-train or rest	Speedwork: Run for 10 minutes 5 × 400 m / 30-second walking or jogging break in between. Run for 15 minutes.	Rest	Cross-train	4.0 miles	Rest	5.5 miles
WEEK 8						
Cross-train or rest	Speedwork: Run for 10 minutes 6 × 400 m / 30-second walking or jogging break in between. Run for 15 minutes.	Rest	Cross-train	4.0 miles	Rest	6.0 miles

Monday	Tuesday	Wednesday	Thursday	Friday	Saturday	Sunday
WEEK 9						
Cross-train or rest	Speedwork: Run for 10 minutes 6 × 400 m / 30-second walking or jogging break in between. Run for 15 minutes.	Rest	Cross-train	4.0 miles	Rest	6.0 to 7.0 miles, depending on your ability level. Some runners find it mentally helpful to run a little past the race distance prior to the race, but it's not necessary.
WEEK 10						
Cross-train or rest	4.0 miles	Rest	3.0 miles	Rest	Rest	10K Race

Your First Half-Marathon Training Plan

Before starting this plan, you should be able to run four miles with minimal walking breaks. Currently, you should be running at least twelve miles per week and have a minimum of three months of running experience. If you're just getting started, begin with the Start-from-Scratch Walk/Run 5K Training Plan and then progress through Owning the 5K Training Plan and the Your First 10K Training Plan, all detailed earlier in this chapter.

When you follow the Half-Marathon Training Plan, the longest distance you'll run is 11.5 miles, 1.6 miles less than the race distance. When you get into long-distance running, there's a point of diminishing returns. Too much distance before the race increases the risk of injury and puts unnecessary stress on the body. Once you become more experienced with running half-marathons, you can increase your long-run distance so you run the race distance a few times before the big day. But as a newbie, it's wise to hold back a bit—don't worry, you'll still be prepared!

During your long runs, it's okay to take regular walking breaks or even cover the entire distance in a walk/run style. Don't stress about your long-run pace; your pace during long runs will naturally be thirty to ninety seconds slower than during your shorter runs. This is actually a good thing, since the slower pace means you're spending more time on your feet, which will provide an advantage on race day. Your race-day pace will be naturally a bit faster than your long-run pace, simply because you'll be pumped up!

Walk/run intervals are not specifically labeled in this plan; however, you can use the walk/run interval method to train for a half-marathon. Week Four and Week Eight of this plan are step-back weeks, which is when you reduce mileage to give your body and mind a break.

Monday	Tuesday	Wednesday	Thursday	Friday	Saturday	Sunday
WEEK 1						
Rest	Speedwork: Run for 10 minutes 5 × 400 m / 30-second walking or jogging break in between. Run for 10 minutes.	Cross-train	3.0 miles	Rest	3.0 miles	4.0 miles

Monday	Tuesday	Wednesday	Thursday	Friday	Saturday	Sunday
WEEK 2						
Rest	Speedwork: Run for 10 minutes 5 × 400 m / 30-second walking or jogging break in between. Run for 10 minutes.	Cross-train	3.0 miles	Rest	3.0 miles	4.5 miles
WEEK 3						
Rest	Speedwork: Run for 10 minutes 5 × 400 m / 30-second walking or jogging break in between. Run for 15 minutes.	Cross-train	3.5 miles	Rest	3.0 miles	5.0 miles
WEEK 4						
Rest	3.0 miles	Cross-train	3.5 miles	Rest	3.0 miles	Rest
WEEK 5						
Rest	Speedwork: Run for 10 minutes 6 × 400 m / 30-second walking or jogging break in between. Run for 10 minutes.	Cross-train	4.0 miles	Rest	3.0 miles	6.0 miles

Monday	Tuesday	Wednesday	Thursday	Friday	Saturday	Sunday
WEEK 6						
Rest	Speedwork: Run for 10 minutes 6 × 400 m / 30-second walking or jogging break in between. Run for 10 minutes.	Cross-train	4.0 miles	Rest	3.0 miles	7.0 miles
WEEK 7						
Rest	Speedwork: Run for 10 minutes 6 × 400 m / 30-second walking or jogging break in between. Run for 15 minutes.	Cross-train	4.5 miles	Rest	3.5 miles	7.5 miles
WEEK 8						
Rest	3.0 miles	Cross-train	3.0 miles	Rest	3.5 miles	8.0 miles
WEEK 9						
Rest	Speedwork: Run for 10 minutes 8 × 400 m / 30-second walking or jogging break in between. Run for 10 minutes.	Cross-train	5.0 miles	Rest	3.5 miles	9.0 miles

Monday	Tuesday	Wednesday	Thursday	Friday	Saturday	Sunday
WEEK 10						
Rest	Speedwork: Run for 10 minutes 8 × 400 m / 30-second walking or jogging break in between. Run for 10 minutes.	Cross-train	5.5 miles	Rest	3.5 miles	10 miles
Monday	Tuesday	Wednesday	Thursday	Friday	Saturday	Sunday
WEEK 11						
Rest	Speedwork: Run for 10 minutes 8 × 400 m / 30-second walking or jogging break in between. Run for 15 minutes.	Cross-train	6.0 miles	Rest	3.5 miles	11.5 miles
WEEK 12						
Rest	4.0 miles	Rest	4.0 miles	Rest	Rest	Half-Marathon Race

Your First Marathon Training Plan

Before starting this plan, you should be able to run a 10K with minimal walking breaks. Currently, you should be running at least fifteen miles per week and have a minimum of six months of running experience. It's important to develop this base, since consistent running will help ward off injuries when you begin to ramp up your mileage in anticipation of a marathon. If you're just getting started, begin with the Start-from-Scratch Walk/Run 5K Training Plan and then progress through the Owning the 5K Training Plan, Your First 10K Training Plan, and Your First Half-Marathon Training Plan, all detailed earlier in this chapter.

For the First Marathon Training Plan, the longest distance you'll run is twenty miles, 6.2 miles less than the race distance. Don't be nervous—twenty miles is far enough to carry you across the finish line on race day. Higher mileage sets you up for injuries, so it's actually safer not to run the complete race distance before the event. Very few marathon training plans—typically only the advanced plans—will ask runners to run the complete distance before race day. While 6.2 miles seems like a huge gap, you'll have the physical endurance to carry you through the finish line if you follow this plan.

During your long runs, it's okay to take regular walking breaks or even cover the entire distance in a walk/run style. Don't stress about your long-run pace; your pace during long runs will naturally be thirty to ninety seconds slower than during your shorter runs. That's okay—it's a good thing to go slowly—you're spending more time on your feet and reducing your risk for injury. Plus, you don't want to crash and burn during the last miles of your long runs. Your race day pace will be naturally a bit faster than your long-run pace, simply because you'll be pumped up!

Walk/run intervals are not specifically labeled in this plan. However, you can use the walk/run interval method to train for a marathon. Week Five, Week Ten, and Week Fifteen are step-back weeks, which is when you reduce mileage to give your body and mind a break. This plan also includes a two-week taper before the race. Don't be tempted to run extra during this taper period; your body needs the rest to be fresh on race day.

Note that the marathon plan includes four days of running each week and one day of cross-training. Seek out a low-impact form of cross-training—like swimming or cycling—to give your legs a break. It's recommended that you do speedwork only once every two weeks, since speedwork is very hard on your body and must be balanced with your increasing distances.

Monday	Tuesday	Wednesday	Thursday	Friday	Saturday	Sunday
WEEK 1						
3.0 miles	Rest	3.0 miles	Speedwork: Run 10 minutes 5 × 400 m / 30-second walking or jogging break in between. Run 10 minutes.	Cross-train or rest	7.0 miles	Rest
WEEK 2						
3.0 miles	Rest	3.0 miles	4.0 miles	Cross-train or rest	8.0 miles	Rest
WEEK 3						
3.0 miles	Rest	3.5 miles	Speedwork: Run 10 minutes 5 × 400 m / 30-second walking or jogging break in between. Run 15 minutes.	Cross-train or rest	9.0 miles	Rest
WEEK 4						
3.0 miles	Rest	4.0 miles	4.0 miles	Cross-train or rest	10.0 miles	Rest
WEEK 5						
3.0 miles	Rest	4.0 miles	Speedwork: Run 10 minutes 6 × 400 m / 30-second walking or jogging break in between. Run 10 minutes.	Cross-train or rest	5.0 miles	Rest
WEEK 6						
4.0 miles	Rest	4.0 miles	4.0 miles	Cross-train or rest	11.0 miles	Rest

Monday	Tuesday	Wednesday	Thursday	Friday	Saturday	Sunday
WEEK 7						
4.0 miles	Rest	5.0 miles	Speedwork: Run 10 minutes 6 × 400 m / 30-second walking or jogging break in between. Run 15 minutes.	Cross-train or rest	12.0 miles	Rest
WEEK 8						
4.0 miles	Rest	5.0 miles	4.0 miles	Cross-train or rest	13.1 miles	Rest
WEEK 9						
4.0 miles	Rest	5.0 miles	Speedwork: Run 10 minutes 6 × 400 m / 30-second walking or jogging break in between. Run 15 minutes.	Cross-train or rest	14.0 miles	Rest
WEEK 10						
4.0 miles	Rest	6.0 miles	4.0 miles	Cross-train or rest	8.0 miles	Rest
WEEK 11						
4.0 miles	Rest	6.0 miles	Speedwork: Run 10 minutes 6 × 400 m / 30-second walking or jogging break in between. Run 15 minutes.	Cross-train or rest	15.0 miles	Rest
WEEK 12						
5.0 miles	Rest	7.0 miles	4.0 miles	Cross-train or rest	16.0 miles	Rest

Monday	Tuesday	Wednesday	Thursday	Friday	Saturday	Sunday
WEEK 13						
5.0 miles	Rest	7.0 miles	Speedwork: Run 10 minutes 6 × 400 m / 30-second walking or jogging break in between. Run 15 minutes.	Cross-train or rest	17.0 miles	Rest
WEEK 14						
5.0 miles	Rest	8.0 miles	4.0 miles	Cross-train or rest	18.0 miles	Rest
WEEK 15						
5.0 miles or cross-train	Rest	8.0 miles	Speedwork: Run 10 minutes 6 × 400 m / 30-second walking or jogging break in between. Run 15 minutes.	Cross-train or rest	8.0 miles	Rest
WEEK 16						
5.0 miles	Rest	7.0 miles	4.0 miles	Cross-train or rest	20.0 miles	Rest
WEEK 17						
5.0 miles or cross-train	Rest	9.0 miles	Speedwork: Run 10 minutes 6 × 400 m / 30-second walking or jogging break in between. Run 15 minutes.	Cross-train or rest	12.0 miles	Rest
WEEK 18						
5.0 miles	Rest	10.0 miles	3.0 miles	Cross-train or rest	20.0 miles	Rest

Monday	Tuesday	Wednesday	Thursday	Friday	Saturday	Sunday
WEEK 19						
5.0 miles or cross-train	Rest	5 miles	Speedwork: Run 10 minutes 6 × 400 m / 30-second walking or jogging break in between. Run 15 minutes.	Cross-train or rest	10.0 miles	Rest
WEEK 20						
3.0 miles	3.0 miles	Rest	Light cross-train	Rest	Rest	Marathon Race

Part IV

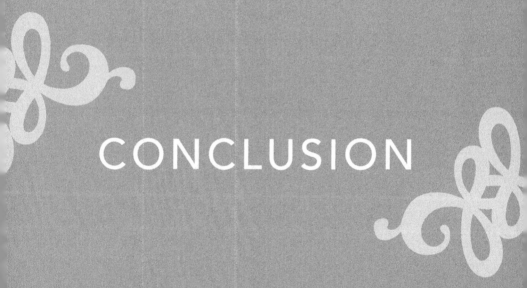

CONCLUSION

YOU DESERVE IT ALL

Health is not a destination. It truly is a lifelong process. By its very nature, health ebbs and flows as we mature and experience life changes. It is my sincerest hope that the *Healthy Tipping Point* has inspired you to view health in a holistic manner; that your mental state is as important as the foods you eat and the exercises you sweat through. Your spirit and body are linked as one. You cannot be truly healthy in body without being healthy in mind. The reverse is, of course, undeniably true.

You *deserve* to be happy and healthy, in spirit and in body. And this transformation begins with just one positive choice. Every single moment is a new beginning. Setbacks only exist until you change your trajectory. If you have a long way to go, don't feel overwhelmed—just focus on your next choice. If you feel like you've fallen off the proverbial healthy wagon, don't stress out—just focus on your next choice. Make your next attitude, next meal, or next workout a healthy, balanced one. These small decisions add up over time and create opportunities for big changes. Over time, your choices become your future.

I hope this book has also inspired you to reconsider what it means to be balanced. Balance does not mean perfection. Maybe your current life circumstances call for cutting yourself a little slack. Maybe you need to push yourself a little harder. Maybe you need to do *less*. Maybe you need to throw a little *more* of your heart into the things you already do. Balance means different things to different people at different times in their lives. When we look at health as a dynamic, holistic aspect of our life, we remove the pressure to be "perfect," and that, my friend, is when truly amazing things begin to happen.

It is never, ever too late to change your life. Perhaps the life of your dreams has been locked within you this whole time, hidden from view because you just haven't acknowledged your own power yet. The life you want is yours for the taking. All you have to do is choose it.

Choose to be happy. Choose to be healthy. Choose the life you want, every day, over and over again.

Acknowledgments

As I sit down to write these acknowledgments, all I can think about is how I never thought *anyone* (besides my mom) would read HealthyTippingPoint.com. Three years ago, I was simply a woman who wanted to become healthier and needed a space to voice my feelings. I owe a huge thank-you to the other bloggers in the healthy living blog genre, as well as to my wonderful readers. Thank you for believing in me and in Healthy Tipping Point. No one achieves success without the help of others, and I will be forever grateful for your support.

I also owe a great deal to Kristien, who was always willing to cook dinner *and* wash the dishes so I could write. Hugs to Mom and Dad for always believing in me.

A huge thanks to Rebecca Scritchfield, MA, RD, ACSM, health fitness specialist. Based in Washington, D.C., Rebecca is a registered dietitian specializing in healthy weight management and behavior change without dieting. Through her products, counseling, and media appearances, she helps people discover the secrets to wellness—food, movement, and fun. Rebecca's advice and suggestions were instrumental in creating the "Eat Clean" section of this book. You can follow Rebecca online at www.rebeccascritchfield.com and @ScritchfieldRD on Twitter.

Also, thanks to Diana from www.thechiclife.com, Jen from www.peanut butterrunner.com, and Victoria from www.novasynchro.net for helping craft the exercise suggestions in "Embrace Strength." Your advice and feedback were invaluable. Kudos to Kath Younger of www.katheats.com and Tina Haupert of www

.carrotsncake.com for being supportive blog friends (blends, shall we say?). Kath and Tina are always willing to guide and support me. You're the blog big sisters I always wanted.

Thanks to Miriam Rich for being a smart and kind editor. And last, thanks to Chris Park for believing in me from the start and helping to make this dream a reality.

Notes

1 Y. Zhang and A. Fishbach, "Counteracting Obstacles with Optimistic Predictions," *Journal of Experimental Psychology: General*, February 2010, accessed June 2011, http://www.ncbi.nlm .nih.gov/pubmed/20121310.

2 Rome Neal, "Caffeine Nation," *CBS News*, February 11, 2009, accessed June 2011, http:// www.cbsnews.com/stories/2002/11/14/sunday/main529388.shtml.

3 "Fat Talk Free Week," Tri Delta, last modified October 10, 2008, http://www.youtube.com/ watch?v=RKPaxD61lwo.

4 Rome Neal, "Healthy Manhattan: Aneroxia Is Not Just for Girls," *New York Press*, June 8, 2011, accessed June 2011, http://www.nypress.com/article-22512-healthy-manhattan-anorexia -is-not-just-for-girls.html; "Eating Disorders in Boys and Men," EatingDisordersHelpGuide .com, accessed June 2011, http://www.eatingdisordershelpguide.com/males-boys.html.

5 Maureen Dowd, "Mama Hugs Iowa," *New York Times*, January 31, 2007, accessed June 2011, http://query.nytimes.com/gst/fullpage.html?res=9C03EED6143FF932A05752C0A96 19C8B63.

6 P.T. Katzmarzyk and C. Davis, "Thinness and Body Shape of *Playboy* Centerfolds from 1978 to 1998," *International Journal of Obesity*, 25, no. 4 (2001), accessed June 2011, http://www .nature.com/ijo/journal/v25/n4/full/0801571a.html.

7 "Eating Disorders: Body Image and Advertising," A Healthy Pace, December 11, 2008, accessed June 2011, http://www.healthyplace.com/eating-disorders/main/eating-disorders-body-image -and-advertising/menu-id-58.

8 "Steps to a New You Improves Size Acceptance/Body Image," *Impact*, May 2008, accessed June 2011, http://www.extension.uidaho.edu/impacts/Pdf_08/5-08mspencer-steps.pdf; "Arnold Schwarzenegger," Body Building Universe, accessed June 2011, http://www.bodybuildin guniverse.com/arnold.htm.

9 Christin Heidemann, DrPH, MSc; Matthias B. Schulze, DrPH; Oscar H. Franco, MD, DSc, PhD; Rob M. van Dam, PhD; Christos S. Mantzoros, MD, DSc; and Frank B. Hu, MD, PhD,

"Dietary Patterns and Risk of Mortality from Cardiovascular Disease, Cancer, and All-Causes in a Prospective Cohort of Women," American Heart Association, July 2008, accessed June 2011, http://www.ncbi.nlm.nih.gov/pmc/articles/PMC2748772/?tool=pmcentrez.

10 Geoffrey C. Ward and Ken Burns, *SuperHealth: 6 Simple Steps, 6 Easy Weeks, 1 Longer, Healthier Life* (New York: Dutton, 2009).

11 "Dietary Guidelines for Americans 2010," U.S. Department of Agriculture, U.S. Department of Health and Human Services, 2010, accessed July 2011, http://www.cnpp.usda.gov/Publications/DietaryGuidelines/2010/PolicyDoc/PolicyDoc.pdf.

12 Ibid.

13 Matt Frazier, "Vegetarian Protein Foods," No Meat Athlete, accessed in July 2011, http://www.nomeatathlete.com/vegetarian-protein.

14 "Soy," BreastCancer.org, April 14, 2011, accessed January 17, 2012, http://www/breastcancer.org/tips/nutrition/reduce_risk/foods/soy.jsp.

15 Amy Myrdal Miller, MS, RD, "To Rinse or Not to Rinse," The Bean Institute, accessed in July 2011, http://beaninstitute.com/recipes/to-rinse-or-not-to-rinse.

16 Susan Thys-Jacobs, MC; Paul Starkey, MD; Debra Bernstein, PhD; Jason Tian, PhD; and the Premenstrual Syndrome Study Group, "Calcium Carbonate and the Premenstrual Syndrome: Effects on Premenstrual and Menstrual Symptoms," *American of Journal Obstetrics and Gynecology*, August 1998, accessed July 2011, http://www.gotmilk.com/pdf/PMSstudy_s.pdf.

17 Michael F. Holick, "Health Benefits of Vitamin D and Sunlight: a D-bate," *Nature Reviews Endocrinology* 7 (February 2011): 73–75, http://www.nature.com/nrendo/journal/v7/n2/full/nrendo.2010.234.html.

18 Deborah Kotz, "Time in the Sun: How Much Is Needed for Vitamin D?" *U.S. News and World Report*, June 23, 2008, accessed in August 2011, http://health.usnews.com/health-news/family-health/heart/articles/2008/06/23/time-in-the-sun-how-much-is-needed-for-vitamin-d.

19 "Seeds, Flax," Self Nutrition Data, accessed August 2011, http://nutritiondata.self.com/facts/nut-and-seed-products/3163/2.

20 "Method 'Green' Household Cleaners Try to Take Market Share from Clorox," Environmental Leader, March 10, 2010, accessed August 2010, http://www.environmentalleader.com/2010/03/10/method-green-household-cleaners-try-to-take-market-share-from-clorox.

21 "Cage-Free vs. Battery-Cage Eggs: Comparison of Animal Welfare in Both Methods," The Humane Society, September 1, 2009, accessed August 2011, http://www.humanesociety.org/issues/confinement_farm/facts/cage-free_vs_battery-cage.html.

22 "Quick Fact," Pesticide Action Network, accessed August 2011, http://www.panna.org.

23 "How Much Is Too Much?" Pesticide Action Network, accessed August 2011, http://www.whatsonmyfood.org/howmuch.jsp.

24 Chensheng Lu, Kathryn Toepel, Rene Irish, Richard A. Fenske, Dana B. Barr, Roberto Bravo, "Organic Diets Significantly Lower Children's Dietary Exposure to Organophosphorus Pesticides," Environmental Health Perspective, 114, no. 2 (February 2006), accessed August 2011, http://ehp03.niehs.nih.gov/article/fetchArticle.action?articleURI=info:doi/10.1289/ehp.8418.

25 Gardiner Harris, "Administration Seeks to Restrict Antibiotics in Livestock," *The New York Times*, July 13, 2009, accessed August 2011, http://www.nytimes.com/2009/07/14/health/policy/14fda.html.

26 James E. McWilliams, "Food That Travels Well," *The New York Times*, August 6, 2007, accessed August 2011, http:www.nytimes.com/2007/08/06/opinion/06mcwilliams.html; Wendy Priesnitz, "Counting Our Food Miles," *Natural Life Magazine*, November/December 2007, accessed August 2011, http://www.life.ca/wendy/articles/foodmiles.html.

27 Sean Poulter, "Why Frozen Vegetables Are Fresher Than Fresh," *Daily Mail*, March 5, 2010, accessed August 2011, http://www.dailymail.co.uk/health/article-1255606/Why-frozen-vegetables-fresher-fresh.html#ixzz1QyRAkfil.

28 "Press Notes," *Food, Inc.* accessed August 2011, http://www.foodincmovie.com/img/down loads/Press_Materials.pdf.

29 Ibid.

30 Mark Bittman, "Rethinking the Meat Guzzler," *The New York Times*, January 27, 2008, accessed August 2011, http://www.nytimes.com/2008/01/27/weekinreview/27bittman.html.

31 David N. Cassuto, "The CAFO Hothouse: Climate Change, Industrial Agriculture and the Law," Animals and Society Institute Policy Paper, 2010, accessed August 2011, http://www .plane taverde.org/artigos/arq_12_05_09_16_09_10.pdf.

32 Bittman, "Rethinking the Meat Guzzler."

33 Ibid.

34 Shigeyuki Muraki, Seizo Yamamoto, Hideaki Ishibashi, Hiroyuki Oka, Noriko Yoshimura, Hiroshi Kawaguchi, and Kozo Nakam, "Diet and Lifestyle Associated with Increased Bone Mineral Density: Cross-Sectional Study of Japanese Elderly Women at an Osteoporosis Outpatient Clinic," *Journal of Orthoapaedic Science*, 12 (2007):317–320, accessed August 2011, http://www.cof.cn/pdf/2007/10/Diet%20and%20lifestyle%20associated%20with.pdf.

35 "How Much Physical Activity Do Adults Need?," Centers for Disease Control and Prevention, accessed August 2011, http://www.cdc.gov/physicalactivity/everyone/guidelines/adults .html.

36 "Virtual Workout Partners Spur Better Results, Study Finds," Science Daily, May 18, 2011, accessed August 2011, http://www.sciencedaily.com/releases/2011/05/110518161707.htm.

37 Jacqueline Stenson, "Another Hurdle to Exercise: Embarrassment," MSNBC.com, December 6, 2006, accessed August 2011, http://www.msnbc.msn.com/id/15598063/ns/health-fitness/t/another-hurdle-exercise-embarrassment.

38 "2011 Marathon, Half-Marathon and State of the Sport Reports," *Running USA*, March 16, 2011, accessed September 2011, http://www.runningusa.org/node/76115.

39 Joanna Scurr, "Bouncing Breasts; a Credible Area of Scientific Research," *Sport and Exercise Scientist* 13 (September 2007), accessed September 2011, http://www.port.ac.uk/departments/academic/sportscience/news/supportingmaterial/filetodownload,78831,en.pdf.

40 Constanza Sol, "Impact Forces at the Knee Joint: A Comparative Study on Running Styles," Pose Tech, May 2001, accessed on September 2011, http://www.posetech.com/library/cs-05 -2001.html.

41 Adam Bean, "Running With Music," *Runner's World*, December 2010, accessed August 2011, http://www.runnersworld.com/article/0,7120,s6-240-466—13768-0,00.html.

42 "Health Benefits of Water-Based Exercise," Center for Disease Control and Prevention, accessed September 2011, http://www.cdc.gov/healthywater/swimming/health_benefits_ water_exercise.html.

43 Marc G. Berman, John Jonides, Stephen Kaplan, "The Cognitive Benefits of Interacting

with Nature," *Psychological Science*, December 2008, accessed September 2011, http://pss.sage pub.com/content/19/12/1207.abstract.

44 Jason L. Talanian, Stuart D. R. Galloway, George J. F. Heigenhauser, Arend Bonen, and Lawrence L. Spriet, "Two Weeks of High-Intensity Aerobic Interval Training Increases the Capacity for Fat Oxidation During Exercise in Women," *Journal of Applied Physiology*, April 2007, accessed September 2011, http://jap.physiology.org/cgi/content/abstract/102/4/1439.

45 "2011 Marathon, Half-Marathon and State of the Sport Reports," *Running USA*, March 16, 2011, accessed August 2011, http://runningusa.org/node/76115.

Index

beverages (*cont.*)
  coffee, 43–44, 141
  soda, 92
  tea, 44, 141, 149
  water, 43–44, 147, 259–60, 261
bicycling
  to purchase bicycle, 272
  spin classes, 289–90
blogs, 9
BMR (basal metabolic rate), 124–25
body acceptance
  children's toys and, 56
  complexity of issue, 56–57
  eating disorders, 51, 63–68
  Fat Talk, 52, 60–61
  healthy body statements, 57–58
  Healthy Ideal, 62
  impact of relationships on, 53
  limiting beliefs and destructive thought
    patterns, 58–60
  media messages about beauty, 20, 53–56,
    61–62
  Myth of Someday, 49–50, 52–53
  negative thoughts, 51–52
  Operation Beautiful, 61
  personal standards of self-worth, 57–58
  small steps toward healthy attitude, 58–62
BodyPump workout, 287–89
boiling cooking technique, 190
boundaries in relationships, 79–80
breakfasts. *See also* smoothies
  Basic Banana Oatmeal in the Microwave,
    195
  Basic Banana Oatmeal on the Stove-top,
    194
  Goat Cheese Frittata, 203–4
  Green and Red Quiche Cornbread,
    199–200
  healthy fuel, 44
  Homemade Almond Butter Granola,
    196–97
  Mexican Breakfast Burrito, 195–96
  No-Egg French Toast, 202–3
  Peanut Butter French Toast, 201–2
  quick and simple, 193
  Savory Oats, 198–99
  Sweet Potato Pancake, 200–201
  Toasted Quinoa and Pumpkin Yogurt,
    197–98
breathing deeply, 42, 46, 77
bribery as motivator, 29

broccoli
  Simple Roasted Broccoli, 225
  Warm Roasted Vegetable
    Salad with Caramelized Pecans,
    207–8
brown rice, *in* Southwestern Casserole, 214
Brussels Sprouts, Caramelized, 226–27
Burrito, Mexican Breakfast, 195–96

calcium, 141–44
calories
  counting, 123–24, 258
  daily needs, 123, 125
  empty, 260
  in macronutrients, 122–23
  in plant-based diet, 104–5
  weight and, 123, 124–27, 260–61
carbohydrates
  calories in, 104–5, 122–23
  as fuel for exercise, 256, 259
  high-protein/low-carb diet, 131
  refined versus unrefined, 108–9
Carolina BBQ Baked Tofu, 221
Carolina BBQ Sauce, 224
cauliflower, *in* Better Than Mashed Potatoes,
    228–29
Center for Science in the Public Interest
    (CSPI), 97–100
cheese
  alternatives and substitutes, 143, 192
  BBQ Tempeh Pizza, 211–12
  Beet This Salad with Balsamic Reduction,
    204–5
  Better Than Mashed Potatoes, 228–29
  Goat Cheese and Apricot Pizza, 210–11
  Goat Cheese Frittata, 203–4
  Green and Red Quiche Cornbread,
    199–200
  ½ and ½ Pizza Dough (with Cheese Pizza
    variation), 209–10
  Holy Deliciousness Bean Dip, 231–32
  Refreshing Watermelon Salad with Sweet
    Balsamic Dressing, 206
  Savory Oats, 198–99
  Southwestern Casserole, 214
  for veggie bowl casserole, 215
  Veggie Cheese Bread, 225–26
chia seeds
  Anne's 5-Minute No-Bake Peanut Butter
    Granola Bars, 237–38
  omega-3 fatty acids in, 146

Printed in the United States
by Baker & Taylor Publisher Services